BOVINE SURGERY AND LAMENESS

Second Edition

A. David Weaver
BSc, Dr med vet, PhD, FRCVS, Dr hc (Wars
Professor emeritus, College of Veterinary M
University of Missouri, USA, and Bearsden,

Guy St. Jean
DMV, MS, Dipl ACVS
Professor of Surgery, Former Head, Department of Veterinary
Clinical Sciences, School of Veterinary Medicine,
Ross University, St. Kitts, West Indies

Adrian Steiner
Dr med vet, FVH, MS, Dr habil, Dipl ECVS, Dipl ECBHM
Professor and Head, Clinic for Ruminants, Vetsuisse-Faculty of Berne,
Switzerland

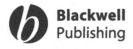

Blackwell
Publishing

Editorial Offices:
Blackwell Publishing Ltd, 9600 Garsington Road, Oxford OX4 2DQ, UK
  Tel: +44 (0)1865 776868
Blackwell Publishing Professional, 2121 State Avenue, Ames, Iowa 50014-8300, USA
  Tel: +1 515 292 0140
Blackwell Publishing Asia, 550 Swanston Street, Carlton, Victoria 3053, Australia
  Tel: +61 (0)3 8359 1011

First published as Bovine Surgery and Lameness in 1986 by Blackwell Scientific Publications
Second edition published in 2005 by Blackwell Publishing Ltd
4   2009

Library of Congress Cataloging-in-Publication Data

Weaver, A. David (Anthony David)
    Bovine surgery and lameness / A. David Weaver, Guy St. Jean, Adrian Steiner. – 2nd ed.
       p. cm.
    Includes bibliographical references and index.
    ISBN 978-1-4051-2382-2 (pbk. : alk. paper)
    1. Cattle–Surgery. 2. Lameness in cattle. I. St. Jean, Guy. II. Steiner, Adrian,
1959– III. Title.

    SF961.W43 2005
    636.089'7–dc22

                                                                      2004028333

ISBN: 978-1-4051-2382-2

A catalogue record for this title is available from the British Library

For further information on Blackwell Publishing, visit our website:
www.blackwellpublishing.com

Contents

Preface to First Edition

This book aims to give the nuts and bolts of practical bovine surgery and lameness.

The text is directed to veterinary students in the clinical years of their undergraduate courses, and to recent and older veterinarians, who experience a limited amount of cattle surgical material. In the interests of compression and simplicity, a single procedure is described in some detail, while the alternatives, known to be equally good in the hands of others, are briefly listed. No apology is made for such dogmatism.

The text includes frequent reference to specific types and sizes of instruments and suture materials. In view of the current move to the metric system, albeit late in the Anglo-American world, all figures are metric, but a comparative scale is included.

All surgery presents a series of challenges, and this accounts for the popularity of the discipline in both the veterinary and medical professions. The challenges in bovine surgery differ from those met by the companion animal surgeon. The first is the economic question: is surgery economically justified? The balance of a judgement to perform a caesarean section on a heifer with dystocia rather than to salvage the animal may be a fine one. This is rarely so in the companion animal field. Humane considerations often complicate an otherwise simple problem.

Other challenges include the anatomical knowledge pertinent to the procedure, the method of restraint and analgesia or anaesthesia, the demands of manual dexterity, and the physical stress imposed on patient and surgeon alike, when surgery must be performed in a sub-optimal environment, which may be the corner of a field or a dark spot in a dusty cowshed.

The inevitable lack of experience in bovine surgery of a young veterinary graduate may persist as a result of a certain apathy among colleagues in the practice group. This apathy is reflected in the difficulties of maintaining equipment necessary for emergency surgery, and results in impatience at the overall time required to complete a bovine operation. The axiom 'time is money' applies as much to the bovine surgeon as to anyone and, since proper instrumentation, asepsis, effective anaesthesia and basic techniques are the keystones to effective craftsmanship, these points are discussed in the first section.

Succeeding chapters logically pass from the head and neck to the abdomen, thence to the female urinogenital system and teat surgery, the male urinogenital apparatus, and finally to lameness. No attempt can be made to treat a subject in depth. The further reading list is similarly selected purely as a basic literature guide.

The reader will often have to consider ethical implications of proposed prophylactic or curative surgery. Animal welfare considerations are becoming increasingly important in many countries. Is castration justified? Is it justified in older cattle, either on humane, economic or management grounds? The relevant veterinary literature is sparse and the conclusions are conflicting. Responsibility rests with the veterinarian.

Why does a farm experience an 'epidemic' of left abomasal displacement cases? The veterinarian may search for further advice on prophylaxis. Such an investigation will often involve other disciplines. A multi-disciplinary approach is particularly needed in herd lameness problems, and the check lists (see pp. 236–238) should stimulate objective recording of herd data and take the emphasis away from repetitive back-breaking treatment of the individual cow.

Serving as a prophylactic, diagnostic and therapeutic instrument, bovine surgery therefore fits into the concept of a herd health programme.

A. David Weaver
Columbia, September 1985

Preface to Second Edition

After an interval of nearly 20 years it seemed appropriate to consider an update. The first edition, translated into 6 languages, appeared to fulfil a need, and a minisurvey of UK veterinarians graduated 2–40 years ago showed unanimous support for such a revision, all emphasising the need for a compact text ('not too many words on a page', 'more simple illustrations') of the standard surgical techniques used in cattle on the farm.

The publishers welcomed the suggestion that two outstanding bovine surgeons, from Switzerland and North America, be invited to add their personal expertise and to provide a wider perspective. As a result this edition has been considerably expanded and has many more line drawings. The style and format have remained strictly instructional, sometimes even dogmatic. Only rarely are alternative techniques discussed, a notable exception being abomasal surgery.

We consider this book should help students in their clinical training, especially when experiencing farm animal practice for the first time, as well as new graduates, inevitably inexperienced, and those veterinarians in mixed practice who may only occasionally be called out for bovine surgical interventions.

More emphasis is placed on animal welfare, for example in suggestions for peri-operative analgesia and anti-inflammatory medication. The authors are all too well aware of the problematic national (EU, other European and North American) regulations on permissible drug usage, and also appreciate that each veterinarian has his or her own preferences.

Effective local, regional or occasional general anaesthesia is demanded today for all painful interventions in cattle. The general public, and not only the involved dairy or beef farmer, also demands that more attention be paid to food safety, and to the replacement of costly therapeutic drugs (often unavailable in developing countries) by prophylactic antimicrobials, and preferably zero drug usage. Such demands necessitate an enhanced need for good antisepsis and sterility.

Surgery may only be carried out when the condition of the patient permits it. The correct decision may be difficult, for example in right-sided abomasal disease, severe dystocia and digital surgery. Economical considerations and farm facilities must also be evaluated in each potential case.

The ever increasing risk over the last 20 years of litigation involving the veterinarian has resulted in more emphasis on the avoidance of potential disasters such as accidental injury to the animal or attendants, or unexpected sequelae to standard surgical procedures. The farm manager or attendant should always be informed beforehand of possible problems, and, we believe, could well occasionally be shown relevant sections of our text on the farm. No veterinarian should undertake any intervention when lacking the necessary confidence or knowledge. We believe bovine surgeons must understand their important role in the worldwide cattle industry today.

The authors trust that this pocketbook will again provide a handy vademecum and a valuable and practical tool in daily practice.

A. David Weaver, Guy St. Jean, Adrian Steiner
February 2005

Acknowledgements

Permission again to reproduce illustrations from the first edition was graciously given by several authors and publishers (Dyce, Pavaux, Cox, Smart), while new illustrations came from several sources as below.

Figs. 1.7, 2.5, 3.2, 3.22 Dr. K.M. Dyce, Edinburgh and W.B. Saunders 'Essentials of Bovine Anatomy', 1971 by Dyce and Wensing

Figs. 2.4, 2.9, 3.1, 3.4, 3.5 Professor Claude Pavaux, Toulouse, and Maloine s.a. editeur from 'Colour Atlas of Bovine Anatomy: Splanchnology' 1982

Fig. 3.15, Dr. John Cox, Liverpool, and Liverpool University Press 'Surgery of the Reproductive Tract in Large Animals' 1981

Fig. 3.24, Dr. M.E. Smart, Saskatoon and Veterinary Learning Systems, Yardley, PA, USA from 'Compendium of Continuing Education for the Practicing Veterinarian' 7, S327, 1985

Fig. 3.17, Dr. H. Kümper, Giessen and Blackwell Science from 'Innere Medizin und Chirurgie des Rindes' 4e 2002 edited by G. Dirksen, H-D. Gründer and M. Stöber fig. 6.125)

Fig. 4.6, Dr. R.S. Youngquist, Columbia, Missouri and W.B. Saunders from 'Current Therapy in Large Animal Theriogenology' 1997 (fig. 57.2)

Fig. 7.12, Dr. M. Steenhaut, Gent, and Blackwell Science from 'Innere Medizin und Chirurgie des Rindes' 4e 2002 edited by G. Dirkson, H-D. Gründer and M. Stöber (fig. 9.159)

Jan Huckin, Newbury, produced many new illustrations from rough sketches by the first author, as did also Don Connor in Missouri. Many others come from the hand of Eva Steiner. John Sprout, Castle Douglas, not only commented usefully on the entire manuscript but also supplied some excellent sketches (Figs. 1.14, 1.15 and 2.2)

Several practising veterinarians have given useful advice including Keith Cutler (Immobilon), Simon Bouisset of Toulouse (analgesics and anti-inflammatories), Bob Miller of Columbia, Missouri, Rupert Hibberd, David Noakes, David Ramsay, and Jan Downer. David Pritchard (DEFRA) and Vincent Molony (Edinburgh) advised on certain aspects of animal welfare legislation pertinent to the UK situation. The RCVS Library helped with some literature sources, and David Taylor checked on the ever-changing microbiological nomenclature, while Lesley Johnson (Veterinary Medicines Directorate) commented on several contentious tables in chapter 1. Appendix 4 was critically assessed for accuracy by Maureen Aitken, Newbury.

The entire manuscript was typed by Christina McLachlan of Milngavie, who deserves thanks for both her accuracy and patience.

Finally thanks are given to all at Blackwell Publishing for their cooperation and advice, including Susanna Baxter, Samantha Jackson, Sophia Joyce, Emma Lonie, Sally Rawlings and Antonia Seymour, also to their copy-editor Liz Ferretti.

Guy St. Jean thanks his mentors Bruce Hull, Michael Rings and Glen Hoffsis, not only for their earlier advice and encouragement during his residency, but also for their continuing friendship. He also thanks Kim Carey for secretarial help and his wife Kathleen Yvorchuk-St. Jean for continual support. Adrian Steiner would like to dedicate the book to Christian.

A. David Weaver, Guy St. Jean and Adrian Steiner,
April 2005

The authors have made every effort to ensure that drugs, their dosage regimes and withdrawal periods are accurate at the time of publication. Nevertheless, readers should check the product information provided by the manufacturer of each drug before its use or prescription.

Drug authorisation by regulatory authorities varies from country to country, and drug withdrawal times, dependent on maximum residue limits (MRL), which are derived from residue depletion studies, can also vary from a parent (proprietary) product to a generic equivalent. Withdrawal times vary within member states of the EU, North America and elsewhere in the world (shown in Table 1.15).

The reader should exercise individual judgement in coming to a clinical decision on drug usage, bearing in mind professional skill and experience, and should at all times remain within the regulatory framework of the country.

CHAPTER 1

General considerations and anaesthesia

1.1 Instrumentation

Instruments should be maintained in good condition and, for common procedures, in sterile surgical packs (caesarean section, laparotomy, teat surgery, orthopedic surgery).

Sterilisation

Instruments should preferably be sterilised by one of the first two methods listed below:

- **autoclaving** by steam, 750 mm/Hg at 120°C for 15 minutes or at 131°C for three minutes for non-packed instruments, or for a shorter time in high vacuum or high pressure autoclaves; 30 minutes for packs at 120°C, or 11 minutes at 134°C.
- **gas sterilisation** by ethylene oxide followed by air drying for several days to avoid diffusion of residual gases from the materials into animal tissues – some acrylic plastic materials, polystyrene and certain lensed instruments may be damaged during this process. Note that ethylene oxide is cancerigenic.
- **cold (chemical) sterilisation** in commercially available solutions, however prolonged immersion is necessary. Health and safety problems exist with products such as glutaraldehyde (Rapidex® Arnolds Vet).
- **simple boiling** of instruments is a poor, slow and tiresome means of sterilisation particularly liable to cause damage. The minimal period of boiling is 30 minutes, longer at altitudes over 300 m. Addition of alkali

Table 1.1   Suitability of various surgical materials for sterilisation.

	Dry heat	Autoclave	Boiling water	Ethylene oxide	Liquid chemicals
PVC (e.g. endotracheal tubes)	no	yes	yes	yes	doubtful
Polypropylene (e.g. connectors)	no	yes	yes	yes	yes
Polyethylene (e.g. catheters, packing film)	no	no	yes* no†	yes	yes
Nylon (e.g. i.v. cannulae)	no	yes	yes	no	doubtful
Acrylic (e.g. perspex)	no	no	doubtful	yes	yes
Silicon rubber	yes	yes	yes	yes	doubtful

*high density
†low density

Table 1.2   Efficiency of different methods of sterilisation.

	Bacteria	Dry spores	Moulds	Fungi	Viruses
Autoclaving	+	+	+	+	+
Gas sterilisation	+	+	+	+	+
Chemical antiseptics	+	—	+	(+)	+
Boiling	+	—	+	+	+

Abbreviations: + = effective; (+) = limited efficacy; — = not effective

to the steriliser increases bactericidal efficiency and boiling time may be safely reduced to 15 minutes. Corrosion is avoided by the addition of 0.5–1% washing soda (Na_2CO_3), while accumulation of lime in serrations or joints is removed by leaving instruments in 5% acetic acid overnight, then brushing off.

Basic instruments for caesarean section or laparotomy

The following is a suggested list of equipment to cover most eventualities.

- towel clamps (Backhaus) × 4, 8.8 cm
- haemostatic forceps (Spencer Wells) × 4 straight 15.2 cm, (Criles) × 2 curved 14 cm, (Halsted) × 2 mosquito straight 12.7 cm

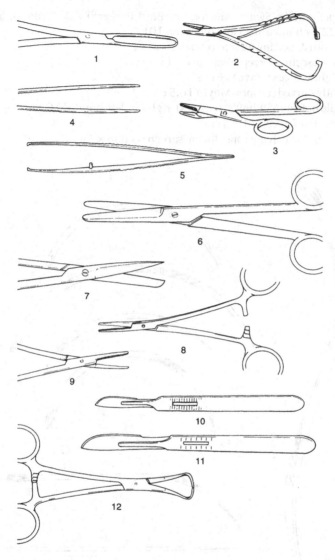

Figure 1.1 Basic instruments for caesarean section or laparotomy.
1. Allis tissue forceps; 2. McPhail's needle holder; 3. Gillies combined scissors and needle holder; 4. plain forceps; 5. rat tooth forceps; 6. Mayo scissors (blunt/blunt), slightly curved; 7. Mayo scissors (pointed/blunt), straight; 8. straight haemostatic forceps; 9. curved haemostatic forceps; 10. scalpel handle no. 4 and no. 22 blade; 11. scalpel handle no. 3 and no. 10 blade; 12. towel clip (Backhaus).

- scalpel handle (Swann-Morton® or Bard-Parker®) × 2, P (no. 4, blades no. 22, or handle no. 3 and blade no. 10)
- rat tooth dissecting forceps (Lane) 15.2 cm
- plain dissecting forceps (Bendover) 15.2 cm
- straight scissors (Mayo) 16 cm
- slightly curved scissors (Mayo) 16.5 cm
- needle holder (McPhail's or Gillies), right- or left-handed 16 cm
- Allis tissue forceps × 4, 15 cm
- sterile nylon calving ropes for caesarean section × 4

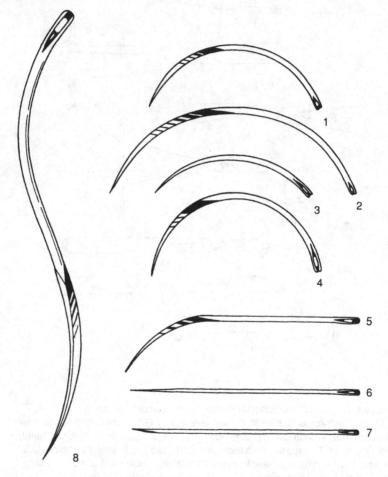

Figure 1.2   Suture needles (shown full scale).
1. and 2. 3/8 circle cutting-edged 4.7 and 7 cm; 3. 3/8 circle round-bodied (taper cut) 4.5 cm; 4. 1/2 circle cutting-edged 4.6 cm; 5. 1/2 curved cutting-edged 6.7 cm; 6. intestinal straight round-bodied (Mayo) 6.3 cm; 7. straight cutting-edged (Hagedorn) 6.3 cm; 8. double-curved postmortem needle 12.5 cm.

- embryotomy finger knife (for incision into uterine wall which cannot be brought near body wall)

Also needed are suture needles, which should include two each of the following types and sizes (see Figure 1.2):

- 3/8 circle cutting-edged 4.7 cm and 7.0 cm
- 3/8 circle round-bodied (taper cut) 4.5 cm
- 1/2 circle cutting-edged 4.6 cm
- 1/2 curved cutting-edged 6.7 cm
- swaged-on curved round-bodied needle 4.5 cm
- intestinal straight round-bodied (Mayo) 6.2 cm
- straight cutting-edged (Hagedorn) 6.3 cm
- double-curved post-mortem needle 12.5 cm

1.2 Asepsis

Bovine surgery involving regions where adequate skin preparation is feasible (i.e. with avoidable microbial contamination of tissues or sterile materials) should be performed under aseptic conditions. Instruments and cloths should be sterile.

Preparation of operative field (e.g. flank):

- close clip wide area, minimum 60 cm cranial-caudal and 90 cm vertically (preferable to shaving)
- alternatively shave operative field after application of disinfectant, soap and water (Schick model razor is suitable)
- wash area with soap and water twice, then scrub with povidone-iodine solution (e.g. Betadine®, [Purdue Frederick], Pevidine, C Vet, Proviodine®, [Rougier]), dry off, wash with 70% alcohol and rescrub
- repeat this procedure three times before respraying with diluted povidone-iodine solution
- large impervious sterile towels, or disposable drapes (rubber or plastic) are useful for placing on the site
- place sterile towel on suitable flat surface for instruments, use sterilised gauze swabs, instruments and suture materials, and sterile gloves

Hand disinfection ('scrubbing up')

Hands are kept in contact with the disinfectant for at least five minutes. Effective hand sterilisation procedures include:

- chlorhexidine 'scrub' (Novasan [Fort Dodge] or Vlexascrub [Vetus])
- 0.5% chlorhexidine concentrate in 90% ethyl alcohol with 1% glycerine as emollient (cheapest), in which 10 ml is first applied to clean dry hands and permitted to dry, before further application and five minutes' scrub-up

Table 1.3 Properties of three common antiseptic compounds.

Generic name	Povidone-iodine	Chlorhexidine gluconate or acetate	Benzalkonium chloride
Proprietary name	Pevidine®, Iodovet® Povidone® (Berk) Betadine® (Purdue Frederick)	Savlon® (Schering-Plough) Nolvasan® (Fort Dodge) Chlorhexidine (Butler, Aspen)	Marinol® (Berk) Zephiran® (Winthrop)
Bactericidal	+	+	(+)
Fungicidal	+	+	+
Virucidal	+	—	—
Dilution			
instruments	undiluted (5%, 7.5% or 10%)		10% diluted 1:500
skin ('scrub')	undiluted (0.75%)	4% or 15 ml of 7.5% solution + 485 ml of 70% alcohol	10% diluted 1:100
wound lavage	0.1%	0.05%	—
Disadvantages	brown skin when dry	incompatible with soap and anionic detergents	incompatible with soap and anionic detergents; fails to kill spore-bearing organisms
Advantages	not inactivated by organic matter	not inactivated by organic matter	—

Abbreviations: + = active; (+) = limited activity; — = no activity

- commercially available povidone-iodine soap
- hexachlorophane suspension applied first dry then wet, but after scrub up (5 minutes) must be fully rinsed off (pHisoHex®, Zalpon)
- sterile surgical gloves should be worn whenever practicable

1.3 Sutures and suturing

Few topics produce such outspoken opinions and dogma as the 'best' suture material and pattern for specific surgical procedures in domestic animals, including cattle. Suture materials are constantly being improved and new products come onto the veterinary market at regular intervals (see Tables 1.4 (a) and (b) and 1.5). This section selects a limited number of materials and methods of usage, and attempts to justify the selection. In few cases can the cost of the material be considered an important factor in selection.

Table 1.4(a) Equivalent gauges for suture materials (metric gauge in this text).

Metric (also Ph. Eur. = European Pharmacopoe)	BP	USP
1	5/0	5–0 (6–0)
1.5	4/0	4–0 (5–0)
2	3/0	3–0 (4–0)
2.5	2/0	—
3	0 (3/0)	2–0 (3–0)
3.5	–(2.0)	0 (2–0)
4	1 (0)	1 (0)
5	2 or 3 (1)	2 (1)
6	3 or 4 (2)	3 & 4 (2)
7	5 (3)	5 (3)
8	6 (4)	6 (4)
9	7 (5)	7 (–)
10	8 (6)	8 (–)
11	9 (7)	9 (–)
12	10 (8)	10 (–)

Values for absorbable suture materials (e.g. multifilament polyglactin 910 [Vicryl] catgut and collagen) are given in brackets
Multifilament polyglycolic acid or PGA Dexon, is also classified as non-absorbable in the above table
BP = British Pharmacopoeia USP = United States Pharmacopoeia

Table 1.4(b) Equivalent gauges for hypodermic needles (metric gauge in this text).

Metric mm external diameter	BWG/G UK/North America
2.10	14
1.80	15
1.65	16
1.45	17
1.25	18
1.10	19
0.90	20
0.80	21

Metric internal diameter is 0.05–0.1 mm less than the external diameter above

Suture materials

Non-absorbable suture materials:

- monofilament nylon (e.g. Ethilon) – skin, *linea alba*
- monofilament polypropylene (e.g. Prolene) – skin, *linea alba*

- pseudomonofilament polyamide polymer (e.g. Supramid®) – skin, *linea alba*
- mono or multifilament surgical steel – skin, *linea alba*

Absorbable suture materials:

- chromic catgut – subcutis, muscle, peritoneum, bowel, bladder, uterus, penis
- multifilament polyglycolic acid or PGA (e.g. Dexon®) – bowel, muscle including teat muscularis
- multifilament polyglactin 910 (Vicryl®) – subcutis, muscle including teat muscularis, bowel, bladder
- monofilament polyglyconate (e.g. Maxon™) – subcutis, bowel, teat (except skin) bladder, uterus
- monofilament polydioxanone (PDS) – bowel, muscle including teat muscularis, *linea alba*
- 'soft' gut (Softgut™) – muscle, bowel, teat muscularis

Discussion

Selection of suture material should be based on the known biological and physical properties of the suture, wound environment and tissue response to the suture.

Monofilament nylon remains encapsulated in body tissues when buried, but the inflammatory reaction is minimal. It has great size-to-strength ratio and tensile strength. It is somewhat stiff and is therefore not particularly easily handled, an important point when operating in sub-optimal conditions of poor light and awkward corners, where the surgeon is bent down. Knot security is only fair.

Multifilament polyamide polymer, encased in an outer tubular sheath (pseudomonofilament), has good strength and provokes little tissue reaction unless the outer sheath is broken, but it loses strength when autoclaved. It is therefore usually drawn from a sterile spool as and when required. It is very easily handled.

Surgical steel has the greatest tensile strength of all sutures, and retains strength when implanted. It has the greatest knot security and creates little or no inflammatory reaction. Surgical steel however tends to cut tissue, has poor handling and cannot withstand repeated bending without breaking. It is sometimes used in tissues that heal slowly (e.g. infected *linea alba*).

Of the six absorbable materials listed, chromic catgut is still commonly used, but has been replaced by synthetic absorbable material in cattle practice. Catgut has relatively good handling characteristics, but also the disadvantages of relatively rapid loss of strength in well vascularised sites (50% in the first week) and poor knot security (tendency to unwrap and loosen when wet). The potential minute risk of the transfer of infectious prion material into food-producing animals (e.g. cattle) and thence into the human

Table 1.5 Comparative qualities (graded unfavourable to desirable, + to +++), of nine selected suture materials for cattle.

Generic name (trade name)	Origin	Tensile strength	Knot security	Handling	Tissue reaction	Resistance to infection	Absorption without inflammation after tissue repair	Cost
Absorbable								
Chromic catgut	collagen	(+)	+		+++	+	+	low
Coated braided PGA (PGS), (Dexon Plus®2)	glycolic acid polymer, coated surfactant	++(+)	++	++(+)	++	++	++	high
Polydioxanone monofilament (PDS¹)	polymer of paradioxanone	+++	++	++	+	+++	+	high
Coated braided Polyglactin 910 (coated Vicryl®¹)	glycolic-lactic acid copolymer	++(+)	++	+	++	++	++	high
Monofilament polyglyconate (Maxon®2)	copolymer of glycolic acid & trimethylene	+++	++		+	+++	+	high
Non-absorbable								
Polypropylene monofilament (Prolene®, Surgelene®, Prodek®)	polymerised polyolefin hydrocarbons	+++	(+)	+(+)	(+)	+++	NA	low
Surgical steel	alloy of iron	+++	+++	+	+	+++	NA	low
Monofilament nylon (Dermalon®, Ethilon®, Surgidek®)	polyamide filament	++(+)	+	+	+	+	NA	low
Polyfilament polyamide polymer (Suprylon®, Vetafil®, Braunamid®)	polyamide polymer	++(+)	++	+++	+	++	NA	low

NA = not applicable
[1]Ethicon [2]Davis and Geck

food chain has led to a ban on the use of chromic catgut in some countries (vCJD risk).

Multifilament polyglycolic acid (PGA) has greater strength which is lost evenly, provoking much less tissue reaction than chromic catgut. PGA is non-antigenic, has a low coefficient of friction and therefore requires multiple throws to improve knot security, but is easily handled.

Monofilament polydioxanone (PDS) is very strong, retaining its strength for many weeks (58% at four weeks), is easily handled, has good knot security, and has the sole disadvantage of provoking an initial tissue reaction which recedes during suture absorption.

'Soft' catgut is undoubtedly the most easily handled absorbable material for delicate bowel anastomoses, its quality even exceeding that of PGA, but it is not yet widely available. Plain or soft catgut is absorbed quickly and maintains its strength for a short time. In coming years PDS and PGA are likely to slowly replace chromic catgut, which will retain its place as a general purpose material. Vicryl® in its coated form is very easy to handle, has minimal tissue reaction and tissue drag. It is stable in contaminated wounds. Polyglyconate monofilament (Maxon™) has three times the strength of Vicryl® at day 21 of wound healing.

Suture needles

Suturing can only be performed efficiently with needles which are rust-free, sharp, and strong enough for insertion through the specific tissue. A selection of needles may be conveniently maintained on a rack in a metallic sterile container.

Discussion

Suture patterns are discussed under the specific procedures. Skin under considerable or potential tension at certain sites, such as the vulval lips and peri-anal region (e.g. following replacement of prolapsed uterus, vagina or rectum), is usually sutured with sterile woven nylon tape 3–5 mm diameter.

1.4 Pre-operative assessment

Introduction

Assessment should include numerous factors apart from the physical condition of the subject:

- potential duration of productive life
- insurance status
- surgical risk regarding complete recovery
- future breeding prospects
- pathology of other body systems directly or indirectly related to primary condition

General physical examination is essential before emergency or elective surgery.

Laboratory tests

Under farm practice conditions laboratory tests may not be performed, but the major parameters very simply estimated with minimal apparatus are:

- packed cell volume: microcentrifuge, microhaematocrit apparatus
- total protein: refractometer

Normal haematological and biochemical parameters of cattle are listed in Table 1.6.

In some abdominal conditions (abomasal torsion or volvulus, intestinal obstruction) estimation of plasma electrolytes (e.g. chloride) is valuable in assessing prognosis and calculating requirements for fluid replacement.

Fluid therapy is discussed in Section 1.11, p. 42.

1.5 Restraint

Introduction
Restraint is necessary for:

- administration of drugs for (a) premedication and sedation, (b) infiltration of local analgesic drugs, and (c) induction of general anaesthesia
- examination and minor interferences carried out without sedation or analgesia/anaesthesia
- prevention of movement in surgical intervention

Restraint may involve physical manipulation of tail, head or nares, or involve application of halter and ropes.

Techniques
Physical restraint by stockman includes:

- halter
- nose grip (fingers or nose tongs)
- tail elevation
- skin grip of crural fold

Rope restraint includes:

- hock twitch
- hindlimb elevation by rope above hock and round an overhead beam
- Reuff's method of casting or sidelines

Many forms of cattle crush or squeeze chute are available with excellent head restraint, which are suitable for surgery of the head and cranial neck (e.g. tracheotomy) and of the perineum. (An essential feature of these crushes

Table 1.6   Reference ranges (haematology and plasma biochemistry) in cattle.

	Units	Average (%)	Range (± 2SD)	
Haematology				
Erythrocytes	$\times 10^{12}$/l	7.0	(5–10)	
Haemoglobin	g/dl	11.0	(8–15)	
PCV (haematocrit)	1/l	35.0	28–38	
Fibrinogen	g/l	4.0	(2–7)	
Leucocytes	$\times 10^9$/l	7.0	(4–12)	
Neutrophils (non-segmented bands)	$\times 10^9$/l	0.02 (0.5%)	0–1.12	(0–2%)
Neutrophils (segmented mature)	$\times 10^9$/l	2.0 (28%)	0.6–4	(25–48%)
Lymphocytes	$\times 10^9$/l	4.5 (58%)	2.5–7.5	(45–75%)
Monocytes	$\times 10^9$/l	0.4 (4%)	0.02–0.8	(2–7%)
Eosinophils	$\times 10^9$/l	0.65 (9%)	0–2.4	(0–20%)
Basophils	$\times 10^9$/l	0.05 (0.5%)	0–0.2	(0–2%)
Neutrophil: lymphocyte ratio	—	0.45:1	—	
Plasma biochemistry				
Urea	mmol/l	4.2	2.0–6.6	
Creatinine	µmol/l	100	44–165	
Calcium	mmol/l	2.5	2.0–3.4	
Inorganic phosphate	mmol/l	1.7	1.2–2.3	
Sodium	mmol/l	139	132–150	
Potassium	mmol/l	4.3	3.6–5.8	
Chloride	mmol/l	102	90–110	
Magnesium	mmol/l	1.02	0.7–1.2	
Total protein	g/l	67	51–91	
Albumin	g/l	34	21–36	
Globulin	g/l	43	30–55	
Glucose	mmol/l	2.5	2.0–3.2	
Alkaline phosphatase	iu/l	24	20–30	
AST SGOT	iu/l	40	20–100	
ALT SGPT	iu/l	10	4–50	
Lactate deydrogenase (LDH)	iu/l	700	600–850	
Bilirubin	µmol/l	4.1	0–6.5	
Cholesterol	mmol/l	2.6	1.0–3.0	
Creatine phosphokinase	mmol/l	3.0	0–50	

The above values refer to healthy adult (> 3 years old) cattle, and have been compiled from various sources. Interpretation of possible deviations from the above ranges should consider variations due to the laboratory technique, breed, lactational and nutritional status, and should always be related to the presenting signs and symptoms of the individual or group. Units are given as SI units

or chutes is the ability to release the head rapidly should the animal collapse.) Many are unsuitable for flank laparotomy, caesarean sections or rumenotomy, however manufacturers will modify sides of crushes (lowering horizontal bar and with a greater space between vertical bars) to improve access to the paralumbar fossa. A veterinary practice may find it advantageous to have such a crush available for surgery on the practice premises or to be transported to the farm. Many crushes have poor facilities for the elevation and restraint of hind- or forelimbs for clinical examination and digital surgery. An exception is the Wopa crush, which is excellent for teat and feet surgery. Suitable crushes may easily be made on the farm and tilted either by manual means or by power.

The use of a crush/squeeze chute should never replace adequate analgesia for surgical procedures.

1.6 Premedication and sedation

Introduction
Premedication and sedation (see Table 1.7) have five aims:

- to improve handling and restraint
- to enhance analgesic effect produced by other anaesthetic agents
- to reduce the induction and maintenance doses of general anaesthesia (GA) agents
- to reduce the possible disadvantageous side-effects of anaesthesia
- to promote smooth post-operative recovery

Very few anaesthetic drugs are approved for use in farm animals. Those known to the authors include azaperone, lidocaine, methoxyflurane and thiamylal (USA). Xylazine is approved for use in cattle in Canada and the UK, and acepromazine is also approved for use in cattle in Canada.

Although not approved for use in cattle in many countries (including the USA), several analgesic drugs (e.g. flunixin meglumine, dipyrone 50% and phenylbutazone, in addition to xylazine) are beneficial as adjunct therapy both pre- and post-operatively in cattle with obvious somatic pain and discomfort. Pre-operative use of analgesics reduces the degree of operative discomfort and post-operative pain. For any medication for cattle in the USA it is the veterinarian's responsibility to consult the Animal Medical Drug Use Clarification Act for guidelines for the extralabel use of drugs, and the Food Animal Residue Avoidance Databank (FARAD) for withdrawal times. (See Appendix 3, pp. 267, legal and professional bodies, for contact details of FARAD).

Xylazine (Rompun® [Bayer])

Advantages
Very useful analgesic and sedative. Xylazine also causes muscle relaxation.

Disadvantages
Causes ruminal stasis, increases salivation, and effects of higher dose rate are somewhat unpredictable as animal may or may not become recumbent. Xylazine is unsuitable as the sole agent for minor surgery when more than a

Table 1.7 Activity and dosage of selected analgesic, anti-inflammatory and sedative drugs in cattle.

	Analgesic	NSAID	Sedative	Dosage (mg/kg) i.m.	Dosage (mg/kg) i.v.
Butylscopolamine bromide/metamizole (Buscopan® Boehringer)	+	+	—	5 ml/100 kg²	
Meloxicam (Metacam® Boehringer)	+	+	—	0.5¹	0.5
Carprofen (Rimadyl® LA soln, Pfizer)	+	+	—	1.4¹	1.4
Xylazine (Rompun® 2% Bayer)	+	—	+	0.05–0.3	0.03–0.1*
Diazepam (Valium®)*	+	—	+	0.5–1.0	0.2–0.5
Flunixin meglumine (Finadyne®, Banamine® Schering-Plough)	+	+	—	—	2.2
Acetylpromazine* (ACP® Novartis)	—	—	+	0.03–0.1	0.03–0.1

*not authorised for use in cattle in UK and EU, may only be given 'off label'
¹by s.c. route, not i.v.
²not authorised in lactating cattle

single painful stimulus is anticipated (e.g. unsuitable as method of analgesia in teat surgery; lancing and drainage of large flank abscess is suitable indication). Xylazine is contra-indicated in the last trimester of pregnancy due to its stimulation of uterine smooth muscle (risk of abortion). It may be used if a uterine relaxant is given before xylazine. Xylazine is contra-indicated in extreme heat, as hyperthermia may result. Avoid accidental intra-carotid injection! Violent seizures and possibly temporary collapse are likely.

Dosage and antagonists

For anaesthetic premedication 0.1 mg/kg xylazine i.m., 0.2 mg/kg i.m. for minor procedures in combination with local analgesia. A faster and more predictable effect is seen following i.v. use (not authorised) at 0.1 mg/kg.

Xylazine sedation, analgesia, cardiopulmonary depression and muscle relaxation are reversible. Also xylazine overdosage (e.g. by inadvertent use of the equine preparation) may be antagonised by different drugs including:

- atropine (100 mg s.c.) to counteract bradycardia and hypotension
- doxapram HCl (Robins) or doxapram 4-aminopyridine (Sigma Chemical Company, St. Louis) respectively 1 mg/kg and 0.3 mg/kg i.v. significantly reduces recovery period
- mixture of doxapram (1 mg/kg i.v.) and yohimbine (Sigma Chemical Company, St Louis) (0.125 mg/kg i.v.)
- yohimbine alone (0.2 mg/kg i.v.)
- tolazoline (4 mg/kg i.v.) – fast onset
- atipamezole (Antisedan® [Pfizer]) 0.02–0.05 mg/kg i.v.

Doxapram acts by direct action on aortic and carotid chemoreceptors and medullary respiratory centre, while yohimbine antagonises xylazine sedation by blocking central α_2-adrenergic receptors.

Chloral hydrate

Long established sedative is given orally (30–60 g as 5% solution but bull requires 120–160 g) or i.v. (5–6 g/50 kg bodyweight as 5% solution). The solution is irritant, and perivascular injection is likely to lead to necrosis and severe skin slough. Infusion (total volume about 1 litre for adult cow) should be made slowly via i.v. catheter over a minimal 5 minute period, since narcosis continues to deepen after completion of injection. Chloral hydrate is not an analgesic. Concentrations required to produce general anaesthesia cause severe, possibly fatal respiratory and circulatory depression.

Atropine sulphate

Drug reduces quantity and increases viscosity of saliva. Premedicant dose in adult cow is 60 mg s.c.

Table 1.8   Properties of four local analgesic drugs (all hydrochloride salts).*

Generic name (trade name)	Lignocaine (Lidocaine®)	Procaine (Ethocaine®)	Bupivacaine (Marcain®)	Cinchocaine (Dibucaine®)
Main indications				
surface analgesia %	2–10	NS	NS	0.25
infiltration %	0.5–1	2–3	0.25	0.25–0.5
Nerve block %	2–3	3–5	0.5	0.5
Epidural block %	2–3	3–5	0.5–0.75	0.5
Rate of diffusion	fast	slow	fast	slow
Duration of action	60–90 mins	< 60 min	≈8 hours	≈8 hours
Analgesic potency	+	+	+	+++
Toxicity	+	+	+	++
Tissue irritation	low	low	low	low
Stability at boiling point	?	good	?	?
Cost (low → high: + → +++)	++	+	+++	++
Other properties	good safety margin, no vasodilator	vasodilator, used with adrenalin	—	decomposes if mixed with alkalis

* several of these drugs are not authorised or licensed for use in certain countries, e.g. only procaine is authorised in UK for use in cattle (unless used in cattle not intended for human consumption)
NS = not suitable

1.7 Local analgesic drugs

The four drugs of greatest value today are the hydrochloride salts of lignocaine, procaine, bupivacaine and cinchocaine (see Tables 1.8 and 1.9).

Lignocaine

Lignocaine (Lidocaine/USP) has largely replaced procaine as it has the advantage of:

- extreme stability
- more rapid diffusion
- longer duration of action
- useful surface analgesic activity on mucous membranes and cornea

It is however no longer authorised for cattle in the UK and EU states, as it has no MRL.

Proprietary names include Lignodrin 2% (Vétoquinol), Lignol (Arnolds), Locaine 2%, (Animalcare), Locovetic (Bimeda).

Toxic effects are rarely encountered (e.g. inadvertent intravascular injection); they include drowsiness, muscle tremors and respiratory depression,

Table 1.9 Selected analgesics for cattle.

Generic name	Proprietary name	Dosage (mg/kg)		
		i.v.	i.m.	oral
Ketoprofen	Ketofen® 10% (Merial)	3	3	NS
Carprofen	Rimadyl® (Pfizer)	1.4	NS	NS
Meloxicam	Metacam® (Boehringer Ingelheim)	0.5	0.5[1]	NS
Xylazine	Rompun® 2% (Bayer)	0.03–0.1	0.05–0.3	NS
Flunixin meglumine	Banamine®, Finadyne® (Schering-Plough)	2.2	NS	NS
Phenylbutazone	*various	2–5	NS	4–8

NS = not suitable; * not authorised for cattle use in UK/EU; [1] by s. c. route

convulsions and hypotension. Toxicity depends on the venous concentration, which in turn depends largely on the rate of absorption. Concentrations for cattle are 2–3%, although 1% is probably adequate for infiltration, nerve block and epidural analgesia.

Proprietary products often contain adrenaline (epinephrine) (concentration 1:200 000). Adrenaline prolongs the activity of lignocaine and reduces the possibility of toxic side-effects.

Lignocaine is also available as:

- 1% or 2% gel with chlorhexidine gluconate solution 0.25%, or hydrobenzoates in a sterile lubricant water-miscible base
- aerosol spray (lignocaine 10%) with cetylpyridinium chloride 0.1%
- 5% cream (Xylodase® [Astra]).

Procaine

Procaine (novocaine) largely replaced cocaine, and has in turn been displaced by lignocaine. However procaine may have economic advantages over lignocaine. Proprietary brands include Planocaine®, Novutox® and Willcain®.

Combined with adrenaline hydrochloride, procaine absorption is slow, solutions may be sterilised by boiling and there is minimal tissue irritation. Metabolite para-amino benzoic acid inhibits action of sulphonamides.

Bupivacaine

Bupivacaine, marketed as Marcain® (Astra) with and without adrenaline (1:4 000 000) as a 0.25, 0.5 and 0.75% (plain) solution, has the following properties:

- analgesic potency and speed of action of lignocaine
- considerably longer (× 4) duration of activity
- very well tolerated by tissues
- indicated where prolonged epidural or perineural analgesia is required
- no MRL in EU

It costs considerably more than lignocaine. The product will doubtless find more widespread use.

Cinchocaine and Carbocaine®-V

Cinchocaine (Nupercaine™, Dibucaine®) is more toxic than procaine, but concentrations for epidural block and surface analgesia are lower (0.5%). Other properties include:

- longer analgesia than with procaine
- drug readily decomposed by action of alkalis and therefore syringes and needles should, if not sterile, be boiled in bicarbonate-free water

Carbocaine®-V or Mepivacain (Pharmacia and Upjohn), 2% solution is sometimes used for infiltration and epidural block, is equivalent to lignocaine and has several hours duration of activity.

1.8 Regional analgesia

Regional analgesia is the preferred method of anaesthesia for many surgical procedures in cattle. Its advantages over general anaesthesia (GA) (see Section 1.9, p. 36) include:

- relatively simple technique
- general availability
- minimal apparatus, e.g. syringe, needles and drug
- little risk of toxic side-effects
- safety

Cornual block

Anatomy

Sensitive horn corium is largely innervated by the cornual branch of the zygomatico-temporal division of the maxillary nerve (from cranial V). Caudally a few twigs of the first cervical nerve make a variable contribution to innervation. The cornual nerve leaves the lacrimal nerve within the orbit, passes through the temporal fossa and around the lateral edge of the frontal bone, covered by fascia and thin frontalis muscle. The nerve is blocked a little below the lateral ridge of the frontal crest, about halfway between the lateral canthus of the eye and the horn (bud) base. The cornual artery and vein are close to the site of block.

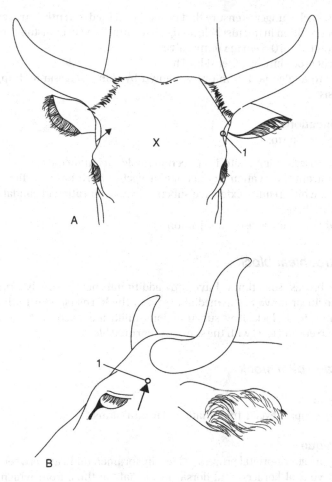

Figure 1.3 Site for cornual nerve block. A. rostral view; B. lateral view; 1 cornual branch of zygomatico-temporal nerve. Note angle of insertion of needle, and also line of cut in skin at horn base in dehorning (see Section 2.1, p. 57). X site on skull for captive bolt euthanasia.

Equipment
Disposable syringe, 10 ml for adults, 5 ml for calves, 2.4 cm 20 gauge hypodermic needle, 2% plain lignocaine or 5% procaine solution (2–8 ml depending on size).

Technique
- insert needle, with syringe attached, midway along lateral edge of crest of frontal bone, directing needle at 30° angle through skin towards horn base (see Figure 1.3)

- draw back plunger to ensure that needle is not inadvertently intravascular
- inject solution in arc just below edge of frontal bone over distance of 1 cm in adults, and 0.5 cm in young calves
- repeat procedure on other side of head
- time to analgesia 3–5 minutes, shown by skin analgesia and upper lid ptosis

Complications
Failures are due to:

- imprecise location of site, i.e. injection made subcutaneously
- significant innervation from caudal aspect to horn base, particularly in bulls, which require extensive subcutaneous infiltration of caudal aspect of horn base
- inadvertent intravascular injection

Infratrochlear block

Exotic breeds sometimes have an additional nerve supply from the infratrochlear nerve to the medial aspect of the horns (similar to that seen in goats). It is blocked by subcutaneous infiltration across the forehead, transversely and level with the site of the cornual block.

Supra-orbital block

Indications
Surgery of upper eyelid, trephination of frontal sinus.

Technique
- palpate supra-orbital process to identify foramen midway between dorsal and ventral borders, and dorsal to medial canthus, from which nerve emerges (branch of cranial V)
- produce insensitive skin wheal over foramen
- insert 1.1 metric 2.5 cm long needle into foramen to depth of 1.5 cm and inject 5 ml of 2% lignocaine (see Figure 1.4)

Alternative technique for regional anaesthesia is local infiltration.

Nerve supply to ocular structures
Innervation of ocular structures is complex:

- eyelids: motor supply – auriculopalpebral branch of facial
             sensory supply – ophthalmic and maxillary branches of trigeminal
- straight and oblique muscles of eyeball: motor supply – oculomotor, abducens and trochlear
- eyeball: sensory – ciliary branch of ophthalmic

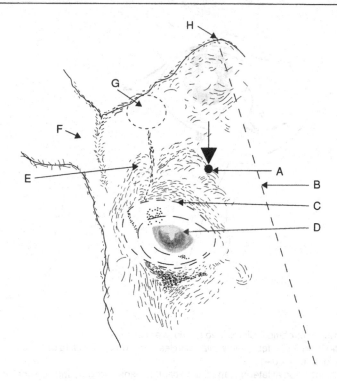

Figure 1.4 Supra-orbital nerve block. Oblique diagrammatic view of right side of head. Foramen is palpable about 3 cm dorsal to upper bony margin of orbit. Long dotted line is midline; dotted line is horn base. A. supra-orbital foramen; B. median line; C. margin of bony orbit; D. orbit; E. frontal bone; F. right ear; G. horn base; H. poll.

The oculomotor, trochlear, ophthalmic and maxillary branches of the trigeminal and abducens nerve emerge from the *foramen rotundum orbitale*.

Retrobulbar block

Indications
- intra-ocular neoplasia (e.g. SCC)
- severe trauma (see p. 68)

Technique
- produce topical analgesia of cornea with butyn sulphate or proparacaine
- insert forefinger into lateral canthus between eyeball and conjunctival sac
- alongside finger pass 1.25 metric 7.5–10 cm curved needle through fornix of conjunctiva until point is retrobulbar (see Figure 1.5)
- ensure that needle point does not enter optic foramen (risk of intrathecal {CSF} injection), and attempt aspiration check

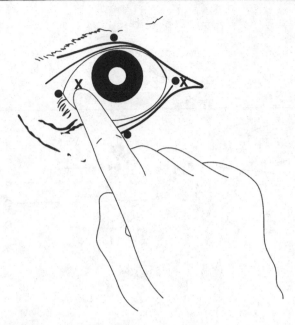

Figure 1.5   Retrobulbar block. Two methods are shown:
(a) needle insertion at four points (black circles) through conjunctiva under careful digital guidance (4 × 8–10 ml);
(b) needle insertion at lateral or medial (×) canthus, again perforating conjunctiva to deposit solution at orbital apex (20–30 ml).
Use 18 gauge needle 15 cm long with marked curvature, advancing tip slowly.

- inject 20–30 ml 2% lignocaine solution, which blocks nerves to ocular muscles causing paralysis of the eyeball and analgesia
- do not attempt to anaesthetise optic nerve, since this may stimulate animal sufficiently to cause fatality
- anaesthetise upper and lower lids by local infiltration as required

Another technique of retrobulbar injection involves placement at four sites (medial, lateral, dorsal and ventral canthi) through the conjunctiva of 10 ml solution at each site, followed by infiltration of the eyelid margins (see Figure 2.8).

Proximal paravertebral block

Indications
Laparotomy, omentopexy, rumenotomy, caesarean section (flank incision); ruptured bladder in calves (midline incision: bilateral paravertebral).

Equipment

Disposable 20 ml syringe, 3 × 1.25 metric 10 cm needles, such as Howard Jones type without stilette, 2% lignocaine with adrenalin. Total volume of solution is 60 ml (three sites) or 80 ml (four sites).

Fat beef cattle may require needle length up to 12–15 cm to reach correct depth.

Technique

- block dorsal and ventral branches of spinal nerves emerging from thoracic 13, lumbar 1 and 2 (for most laparotomy procedures excepting caesarean section) or L1, L2 and L3 (caesarean section alone)
- ensure good head restraint and, depending on temperament of cow, stand on opposite side to that to be blocked, leaning over back
- clip and scrub skin from last rib to *tuber coxae* along a band 15 cm wide, to left or right of dorsal midline as appropriate
- block L2 first: identify its transverse process by counting forwards from last palpable process (L5) which is just cranial to sacral tuberosity of ilium
- locate point (adult Friesian cow) precisely 5 cm from midline and level with caudal lateral edge of L2 transverse process (see Figure 1.6)
- punch needle vigorously through skin and *longissimus dorsi* musculature, directed almost perpendicularly but with shaft inclined 10° medially
- advance needle firmly to contact and pass over caudal border of L2 transverse process, through intertransverse ligament (dense fibrous tissue

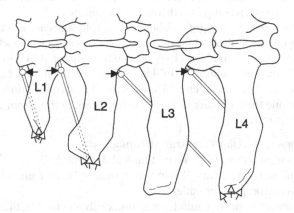

Figure 1.6 Paravertebral anaesthesia: horizontal diagrammatic view of left lumbar vertebrae 1–4 to show course of last thoracic (T13), first three lumbar nerves, and position of needle. Black arrows indicate the direction in which the vertical needle point is 'walked off' the transverse process in the proximal technique. White arrows show the area of infiltration above and below the tips of processes 1, 2 and 4 in the distal technique.

offering momentarily more resistance to needle point) and advance 1 cm further. Needle point now lies where dorsal and ventral branches of L2 spinal nerve have just emerged and separated adjacent to spinal foramen

- attach syringe with 20 ml solution and after applying negative pressure (check needle is not in blood vessel) inject 15 ml solution in an area about 1 cm below ligament, moving shaft and needle point around very slightly
- inject remaining 5 ml solution during first stage of withdrawal of needle above level of ligament to block aberrant dorsal cutaneous fibres
- remove needle while pushing skin down firmly to avoid development of subcutaneous emphysema
- block L1, (see Figure 1.6) site found by measuring distance between two lumbar transverse processes, and again inserting needle 6 cm from midline and directing needle point over the caudal edge of L1 transverse processes
- block cranial site (T13) by advancing needle off cranial edge of L1. Insert needle through skin about 5 cm cranial to previous insertion point. Distance travelled by needle shaft is usually slightly more than for preceding sites
- in case of caesarean section, one may block L3 in similar manner to L2, but omit T13

Field of analgesia

Commencing analgesia is noted by convex curvature of spine (scoliosis) on injection side resulting from relaxation of *longissimus dorsi* and flank musculature. Analgesia is complete within 10–15 minutes.

Field of analgesia runs slightly obliquely ventrally and caudally to midline. Innervation of the individual dermatomes overlaps so that a block of single nerve produces a very narrow (1–4 cm wide) analgesic skin band over the flank. T13 innervates skin over middle of last 1–2 ribs (12–13), while L3 block causes analgesia as far caudal as *os coxae*. Dorsal ramus innervates skin over upper one third of flank skin, the ventral ramus the remainder of the flank (see Figure 1.7).

- T13: dorsocranial flank, ventrally to umbilicus
- L1 (*n. iliohypogastricus*): dorsal midflank abdominal wall
- L2 (*n. ilioinguinalis*): caudal flank skin over stifle and inguinal region, scrotum and prepuce, or udder
- L3 (*n. genitofemoralis*): caudal flank, especially ventrally, stifle, inguinal region, scrotum and prepuce, or udder

Variations of technique have included production of insensitive skin wheal prior to insertion of a longer needle, and insertion of a stout 2.1 mm diameter needle to infiltrate the musculature, later replaced by a finer and longer needle.

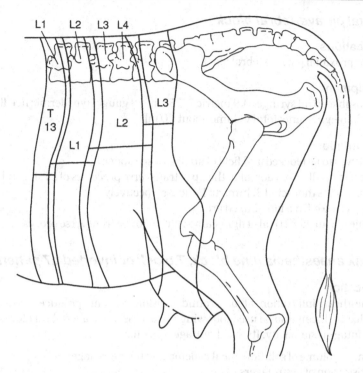

Figure 1.7 Diagram of innervation of left flank: paravertebral anaesthesia. Horizontal bars indicate width of skin analgesia from block of individual nerves. Note degree of overlap of dermatomes and caudal displacement of analgesic field relative to the particular nerve root. (Modified from Dyce & Wensing, 1971.)

Discussion

Block is easier in cattle in poor body condition. Analgesic technique in exceptionally large-framed and fat cattle may require a needle 12 cm long. Successful block results in moderate convexity of the spine on the analgesic side (scoliosis), together with localised hyperthermia.

Block of L4 may sometimes cause mild ataxia. Advantages of paravertebral block over flank infiltration include:

- minimal volume of anaesthetic solution
- absence of anaesthetic solution in surgical field
- large area of desensitisation
- rapid onset of action

Distal paravertebral block

Indications

As for proximal paravertebral block.

Equipment

Disposable 30 ml syringe, 0.9 metric 3.75 cm, 18 gauge hypodermic needles, 2% plain lignocaine; total volume about 60 ml.

Technique

- nerves to be blocked and field of analgesia see above
- insert needle 3 cm dorsal to the tip of transverse processes of L1, L2 and L4 for nerves thoracic 13, lumbar 1 and 2 respectively
- inject 10 ml in a fan-shaped area
- inject a further 10 ml of lignocaine ventral to the transverse process

Flank anaesthesia (line block, T block or inverted L7 pattern)

Indication

Anaesthetic infiltration at or around incision site can produce adequate analgesia. It can also be used following unsuccessful paravertebral block. Its advantage is simplicity. Its disadvantages include:

- large volume of solution, local oedema and haemorrhage
- distortion of tissue layers
- poor analgesia of peritoneum
- poor muscle relaxation
- increased post-operative swelling
- increased risk of wound infection

Technique

- infiltrate subcutaneous tissues, muscularis and the sub-peritoneal layers in three distinct movements
- insert needle at point where horizontal and vertical bars of imaginary 'T' join (see Figure 1.8). This point forms dorsal commissure of intended flank incision
- pass needle (1.1 metric 10 cm) cranially to full extent subcutaneously, and infiltrate with 2% lignocaine (plain) during slow withdrawal
- detach syringe and, without removing needle from skin, direct point caudally and advance, and likewise infiltrate during withdrawal
- repeat with infiltration of deeper tissues (total of about 60 ml in horizontal line)
- insert needle 10 cm ventral to previous point and similarly infiltrate proposed incision line (another 60 ml, i.e. total about 120 ml in adult cow)

Note that needle is only inserted through skin twice in entire infiltration.

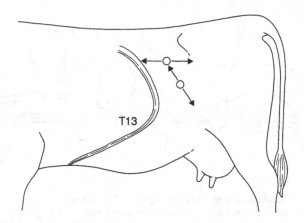

Figure 1.8 Method of infiltration of body wall of flank in 'T block'; technique can also be used in 'reverse 7 block'. Note that the needle is only inserted through skin twice in whole analgesic procedure.

'Reverse 7 block'

A slight variation in the linear infiltration of the flank is the 'reverse 7 block', or 'inverted L block' which are self-explanatory (see Figure 1.8).

Epidural block

Indications

Caudal epidural: intravaginal and intrauterine manipulations (e.g. embryotomy), dystocia (block abolishes tenesmus), replacement of vaginal and uterine prolapse, rectal prolapse, perineal and tail surgery.

Cranial epidural (same site, larger volume of analgesic solution): flank laparotomy, surgery of hindlimbs and digits, penis, inguinal surgery, udder and teat surgery.

Solution is injected into epidural space which caudally contains branches of spinal nerves (*cauda equina*) invested with epineurium (*dura mater*), small dorsal and ventral venous plexuses, and variable amount of fatty tissue.

Equipment

- 10 ml (caudal epidural) or 30 ml syringe (cranial)
- short bevelled 5 cm 1.25 metric needle
- 2% lignocaine without adrenaline
- 2% xylazine

Preparations containing preservatives such as chlorocresol and sodium metabisulphite (e.g. Locovetic [Bimeda]) are unsuitable for epidural injection.

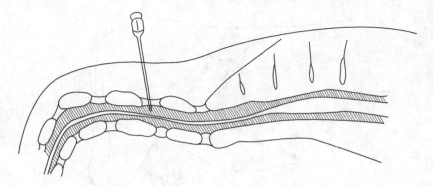

Figure 1.9   Caudal epidural block at coccygeal 1–2 interspace.
s = sacrum; shaded area is spinal canal with *cauda equina*.

Technique

- locate first intercoccygeal space (Co1–Co2) which undergoes significant movement when tail is elevated (sacrococcygeal space is virtually immobile). It measures about 1.5 cm transversely and 2 cm craniocaudally (see Figure 1.9)
- aseptic procedure, so clip site with scissors and disinfect. Entry of infection is a serious problem, and can lead to permanent paralysis of tail resulting in persistent faecal contamination of perineal skin and udder, and subsequent culling
- insert needle precisely in midline, directed very slightly cranially, shaft forming angle of 15–20° with vertical in standing animal. Note structures penetrated are skin, fat and interarcuate supraspinous and interspinous ligaments
- appreciate at depth of about 2 cm that point of needle is freely moveable
- inject 5 ml of lignocaine solution slowly
- an audible sound ('whoosh') may be appreciated

If resistance is encountered, the needle has been inserted too deeply and has entered cartilagenous tissue of intervertebral disc (point cannot be moved from side to side) or, though free in epidural space, needle lumen may be blocked by fibrous tissue. In either case remove needle and repeat with new needle.

Caudal (low) block – dose is 5–10 ml of lignocaine in adult cows, 10–15 ml in bulls, 1–3 ml in calves (approx 1 ml/100 kg). Field of analgesia with caudal block extends from tail base to ventral perineal skin and approximately 25–30 cm lateral to midline. Increased dosage to 30 ml invariably causes ataxia, with recumbency in many individuals.

Cranial (high caudal) block – dose is 40–80 ml in adult cattle, 5–25 ml in calves. Hindlimb function is affected by desensitisation of L6 and sacral (S) 1 and 2 nerves (sciatic supply) L5 and L6 (obturator and femoral) and more cranial nerves. Dysfunction, depending on the degree of involvement, ranges from mild ataxia and slight spasmodic flexion and extension of stifle and hock joints to complete posterior paralysis.

Discussion
Major disadvantage is the risk of injury during onset (ataxia) or recovery phase (e.g. hip dislocation). Recovery to standing takes several hours, and animal should not be permitted to attempt to stand until tail sensation has returned. Keep in sternal recumbency with hind legs roped together above hock, or sedate with xylazine or acetylpromazine to prevent attempts to stand. Consider moving to straw-bedded box or yard.

Factors affecting extent of epidural block include volume, bodyweight, pregnancy and position of cow.

Xylocaine-lignocaine combinations
Analgesia after epidural administration of xylazine (0.05–0.1 mg/kg body-weight of 2% solution, diluted to total volume of 5–10 ml with sterile 0.9% NaCl solution or distilled aqua; alternatively 0.03 mg/kg diluted with 2% lignocaine to 5 ml total volume for adult cow) lasts twice as long (four hours) as after equivalent use of lignocaine HCl (0.2 mg/kg) alone. Very useful in cows with chronic tenesmus (see Section 3.19, p. 138). Extent of perineal anaesthesia is more variable than with lignocaine, but has been reported to include the entire perineal region, including udder and flank. Side-effects include marked transient sedation, hindlimb ataxia, bradycardia and hypotension, and can be reversed by i.v. tolazin (Priscoline HCl, 0.3 mg/kg) without affecting analgesia.

Pudic (internal pudendal) block

Indications
Penile surgery distal to sigmoid flexure, examination of prolapsed penis in standing animal.

Equipment
1.65 metric 12 cm needle, 30 ml syringe.
2% lignocaine

Technique
Larsen method involves block of the pudic nerve (fibres of ventral branches of S3 and S4) and anastomotic branch of middle haemorrhoidal nerve (S3 and S4) via an ischiorectal fossa approach.

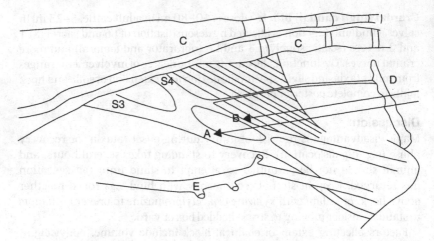

Figure 1.10   Pudic (internal pudendal) nerve block. Diagram shows nerves (from sacral 3 and 4), and injection sites A and B on medial surface of right pelvic wall and floor of cow (pelvic viscera removed).
A. is just dorsal and lateral to sacro-sciatic foramen; B. is slightly more caudal and dorsal; C. sacrum and coccygeal vertebrae 1–3; D. anus through which hand is inserted only to wrist level; E. internal pudic artery (pulsation!) lies just ventral to sites A and B.

- scrub perineal region clean and insert gloved hand in rectum to locate nerve lying on sacrosciatic ligament immediately dorsal and lateral to sacrosciatic foramen, which is less than a hand's breadth cranial to anal sphincter
- note pulsation of internal pudic artery just ventral to nerve
- insert needle forward at deepest point of ischiorectal fossa, directed slightly downwards for a distance of 6 cm (see Figure 1.10)
- check position of needle point by rectal digital control and inject 20–25 ml solution (2–3% lignocaine) around nerve
- inject a further 10–15 ml slightly more caudally and dorsally
- inject 10–15 ml slightly cranially and ventrally, at cranial border of foramen, for more effective block of ventral branch of the pudic nerve
- repeat procedure on other side of pelvis, reversing position of hands

Manipulation of a long needle is easier if a short stout (2.1 metric 2.4 cm) needle is inserted through skin, producing analgesic skin wheal and serving as canula for the longer needle. Alternatively caudal epidural block (5 ml) rapidly desensitises the area of intended needle insertion.

Pudic block is effective after 30–40 minutes, and persists several hours. The main advantage is that subject remains standing, while volume of drug necessary to block nerve supply to penis by epidural technique almost invariably causes posterior paralysis. Cleanliness and experience of the pelvic landmarks are the main criteria for success with pudic block. Technical failures are common in inexperienced hands, and delay before onset of analgesia is a further drawback.

Block of dorsal nerve of penis

The alternative technique to pudic block for penile relaxation and analgesia involves analgesia of the dorsal nerve of the penis as it passes over the ischial arch.

Technique
- infiltrate skin 2.5 cm from midline adjacent to the penile body
- insert needle, advancing to contact pelvic floor and withdraw 1 cm (see Figure 1.11)
- check that needle is not intravascular (dorsal artery of penis)
- infiltrate 20–30 ml 2% lignocaine (plain) into region
- repeat procedure on opposite side of penis

Onset of analgesia in about 20 minutes, duration one to two hours.

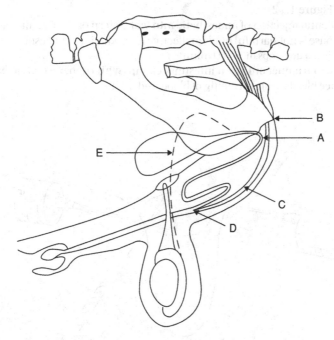

Figure 1.11   Block of dorsal nerve of penis at ischial arch.
A. insertion of needle horizontally 2.5 cm from midline where penile body is palpable below level of *tuber ischii*; B. *tuber ischii*; C. retractor penis muscles and penis; D. point of insertion of retractor penis muscles; E. ductus (vas) deferens.

Teat block

Indications
Teat analgesia is required for repair of teat lacerations (perforating fistula and severe lacerations), polyps, sphincter damage causing obstruction, and supernumerary teats. Analgesia is also needed for teat endoscopy (not discussed further).

Equipment
20 ml syringe, 1.10 metric 2.4 cm needle, catapult elastic and large curved artery forceps.
2% lignocaine

Technique
- inject sedative drug into cow or heifer
- perform local infiltration of teat base after removing any obtruding hairs from udder
- insert needle subcutaneously transverse to direction of teat, and make subcutaneous injection of 10–20 ml solution as a peripheral (ring) block (see Figure 1.12)
- accidental injection of anaesthetic into teat cistern or the circular veins at teat base is not harmful but is ineffective in producing analgesia
- analgesia develops in 5–10 minutes
- place tourniquet or Doyen intestinal clamp (with rubbers) on teat base to reduce bleeding and dripping of blood and milk

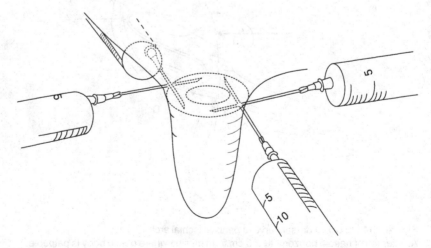

Figure 1.12 Teat ring block: 10–20 ml of 2% lignocaine are evenly distributed around base of teat.

Discussion

Infusion of the teat cistern is not recommended. Even cases of polyps and stenosed teat orifices prove difficult to block in this way because only the mucous membrane becomes desensitised, presumably because subcutaneous and muscularis layers are also involved in the surgical trauma.

The entire teat is anaesthetised distal to the site of injection. An alternative technique is by i.v. injection of any superficial teat vein distal to a tourniquet. This produces analgesia throughout the teat. This technique is virtually only possible in a recumbent cow.

Intravenous regional analgesia of digit

This technique is simple and effective and supersedes the cumbersome local infiltration or nerve block procedures. It is indicated in any painful interference distal to hock and carpus, and is ideal for digital surgery. No tourniquet is required for foot surgery on a cow in a Wopa crush (see below).

Equipment

Tourniquet of stout rubber tubing, metal clamp to fix tourniquet, two rolls of muslin bandages (or similar padding material), 20 ml syringe and 1.1 metric 4 cm needle.

Technique

Cow in lateral recumbency:

- restrain animal in lateral recumbency, preferably after i.v. or i.m. injection of xylazine (0.1 mg/kg) for sedation, with affected limb uppermost
- wrap rubber tourniquet firmly around limb proximal or distal to hock or carpus (see Figure 1.13)
- in hindlimb place a rolled bandage in depression on either side of limb between Achilles tendon and tibia to increase pressure on underlying vessels
- clip (or shave) hair over any convenient and visible superficial limb vein distal to the tourniquet. The lateral saphenous or lateral plantar digital vein is a suitable site in the hindlimb (see Figure 1.13)
- insert 1.10–1.65 metric (16–19 BWG) needle with syringe attached, either in proximal or distal direction, into the vein and inject 20–30 ml 2% lignocaine, with or without adrenaline, as rapidly as possible
- remove needle from vein and massage site well for one minute to prevent development of subcutaneous haematoma
- in forelimb tourniquet is placed around distal radius or proximal metacarpus and make injection into superficial vein medially, e.g. cephalic over distal radius, or medial superficial metacarpal distal to carpal joint over deep flexor tendon

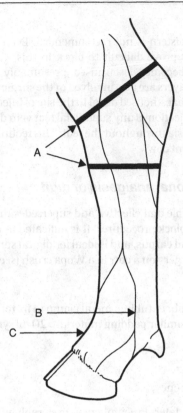

Figure 1.13 Intravenous regional anaesthesia. Lateral aspect of left hind limb of cow showing two possible positions for tourniquet (A) and sites for injection into lateral digital vein (B) and dorsal common digital vein (C, lying deep, at pastern between the proximal phalanges).

Cow standing in Wopa crush:

- elevate limb using strap and buckle, fixed overhead (strap is efficient tourniquet)
- note lateral saphenous vein prominent in proximal quarter of metatarsus (see Figure 1.14)
- push vein sideways to make it more prominent and relatively immobile
- guide loaded syringe proximally towards vein using ball of thumb to steady syringe (see Figure 1.15)
- analgesia develops in entire limb distal to tourniquet after about five minutes and is optimal in ten minutes, persisting for at least 90 minutes if the tourniquet is left in place

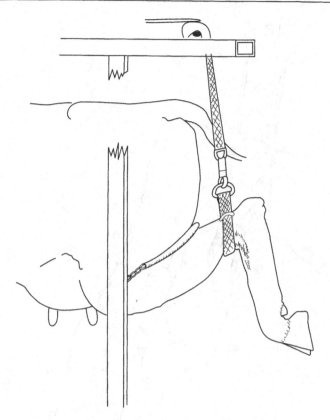

Figure 1.14 IVRA in standing cow in Wopa crush. Strap forms efficient tourniquet to occlude lateral saphenous vein.

Discussion

The speed of onset is governed by the volume, since higher intraluminal pressure causes more rapid diffusion of the solution (e.g. 30 ml versus 20 ml). The tourniquet may safely be left for two hours, although few surgical procedures ever require this length of time. Usually surgery is finished in 10–30 minutes, when the tourniquet may be safely released. Sensation returns within five minutes. Lack of success is generally due to slackness of the tourniquet which has failed to occlude the vascular drainage of some deeper vessels. Analgesia occurs latest in the interdigital region.

Toxic signs have rarely been reported in cattle if the tourniquet has remained in place for over 20 minutes. Signs of toxicity can include drowsiness, minor convulsions and seizures, trembling and profuse salivation with hypotension. Lignocaine is rapidly detoxicated in the liver.

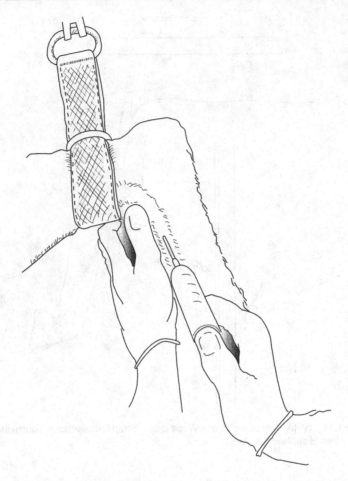

Figure 1.15 Close-up view of injection of anaesthetic solution into lateral saphenous vein. Thumb pushes sideways to fix vein while simultaneously steadying syringe barrel.

1.9 General anaesthesia

Indications

General anaesthesia (GA) is rarely indicated in cattle. It is practised if the usual techniques of regional and local analgesia either cannot be adopted, or fail. Specific indications include extensive surgery of the head, neck, chest and abdomen, as well as the body wall and intra-abdominal experimental manipulations, (e.g. embryo transfer), as well as most long bone fractures when maximum relaxation is desired. GA has a relative surgical indication when complete asepsis is essential, such as in umbilical hernia repair in calves. For GA, food should be withheld for 6–12 hours in calves and for up to 36 hours in adult cattle. Restriction of water is not indicated in calves, and should not exceed 12 hours in adults.

Disadvantages of GA

Risks of GA in cattle include regurgitation, ruminal tympany, poor oxygenation and skeletal injury.

(a) **Risk of regurgitation** and subsequent aspiration of ruminal contents and saliva into the trachea, bronchi and alveoli with potential lethal consequences (necrotic laryngotracheitis and necrotising bronchopneumonia with pulmonary oedema). Endotracheal intubation is therefore essential to avoid this problem.

Factors affecting regurgitation include:
- depth of anaesthesia (see Table 1.10) – light level provokes active regurgitation, deep level passive regurgitation
- degree of ruminal distension or tympany
- fluidity of ruminal contents
- body and head/neck position
- body movement as in struggling and repositioning of animal
- volume of saliva
- duration of anaesthesia

(b) **Risk of severe ruminal tympany** (see above and below).
(c) **Risk of severe compromise** of the effective expansion capacity of lungs as a result of:
- increased abdominal size following development of ruminal tympany causing pressure on diaphragm
- relatively poor oxygenation of the dependent lower lung due to inadequate circulation and pressure (ventilation-perfusion mismatch). Poorly oxygenated blood from ventral lung mixes with better oxygenated blood from upper dorsal lung, giving lowered systemic oxygenation and increased CO_2 retention (hypercapnia).

(d) **Risk of skeletal injury** in induction and recovery, involving possible dislocation, myositis and nerve paralyses.
(e) Expense and size of gaseous anaesthetic equipment, and appropriate expertise in its use.

Equipment

Apparatus for GA of cattle older than three to six months is similar to that available for horses. Endotracheal intubation is essential in bovine GA. Equipment for volatile and gaseous agents is of circle and to-and-fro pattern, incorporating soda-lime canister and re-breathing bag with either an

Table 1.10   Main signs for assessing anaesthetic depth.

	Surgical anaesthesia	Excessive depth*
Cardiovascular system		
Heart rate and rhythm	tachycardia	bradycardia, impending arrest
Muscous membrane colour	pink	cyanotic
Capillary refill time	< 2 sec	> 3 sec
Respiratory system		
Respiratory rate	near normal	shallow, irregular, gasping, apnoea
Tidal volume	slightly reduced	more reduced
Character	regular	irregular
Ocular signs		
Position and size of pupil	moderately constricted, possibly rotated down	very dilated, centrally fixed
Palpebral reflex	present	very slow or absent
Corneal reflex	present	slow
Musculoskeletal system		
Muscle tone		
(lower jaw, limbs)	moderate	poor or absent
Other signs		
Swallowing reflex	absent	absent
Salivary flow	present, profuse	absent
Lacrimal secretion	present	absent

* Action to take in case of excessive depth:
● note time
● check patency of airway
● stop any volatile anaesthetic administration, give oxygen and artificial respiration
● check heart rate (for five seconds)
● check respiratory rate and character (for five seconds)
● check other vital signs (see above)

uncalibrated or calibrated vaporiser (0–5%) to volatilise halothane (Fluothane® [Schering-Plough, Mallard Medical]), isoflurane or sevoflurane) by means of oxygen delivered by a preset flowmeter. Minimum internal diameter of airways in such apparatus should be 4 cm.

Equipment for GA of calves with volatile or gaseous agents is similar to that for larger breeds of dog, e.g. Boyle's circle absorber. The airway diameter, although theoretically inadequate, is unlikely to produce disadvantageous side-effects. Endotracheal tubes for calves should have an internal diameter of 12–16 mm, while those for adult cattle should be about 2.5 cm. Tubes of siliconised PVC are approximately one quarter the price of rubber endotracheal tubes (adult cattle).

List of equipment for GA by gaseous or volatile agents:

- anaesthetic apparatus – circle or to-and-fro system
- endotracheal tubes (calf-adult: 12–25 mm)
- syringe for inflation and clamping-off of cuff
- mouth gag (e.g. Drinkwater model)
- laryngoscope (e.g. Rowson pattern) optional
- nasogastric tube to act as guide, over which endotracheal tube is passed (alternative)
- halothane, isoflurane or sevoflurane and oxygen supply
- ruminal trocar and cannula

Intravenous drugs

Intravenous agents for GA of cattle include:

- **thiopentone sodium** – give as 10% solution by rapid i.v. injection, dose 1 g/100 kg 10 minutes after xylazine premedication or 1.2 g/100 kg if unpremedicated. Perivascular injection is irritant, therefore following such an accident, infiltration of 500 ml saline with hyaluronidase is essential to prevent perivascular necrosis and skin slough. Duration of GA 5–8 minutes. Recover to stand in 30–60 minutes. Unsuitable for very young calves.
- **ketamine and xylazine** – xylazine is given i.v. (0.1 mg/kg) or i.m. (0.2 mg/kg), immediately followed by i.m. ketamine (2 mg/kg).
- **chloral hydrate** – unsuitable for GA of cattle, but remains an inexpensive sedative (see p. 15).
- **ketamine and guiafenesin**: 1 g of ketamine is added to a 1 litre bag or bottle of a 5% guaifenesin solution. This combination is administered to effect at about 0.2–0.5 ml/kg/hour and produces satisfactory anaesthesia which can be maintained for several hours.

In any such intravenous GA technique endotracheal intubation should be carried out as soon as possible after injection. The tube should only be removed following a demonstrable cough reflex or swallowing movement. Extubation is performed with the head lower than the trunk and with the cuff inflated until it reaches the pharynx, preventing material moving between tube and tracheal mucosa, dribbling towards the bifurcation of the bronchi and causing a necrotic bronchotracheitis.

Immobilon™/Revivon™ – large animal product

A reversible neuroleptanalgesia (narcosis) with analgesia can be attained for restraint and surgical procedures with LA Immobilon™, the active principle of which is etorphine, combined with acetylpromazine. It is not licenced for use in cattle, but is sometimes used in exceptional circumstances where other methods of restraint are considered too hazardous. The drug is extensively used in various species in tropical Africa, but rarely now in the UK except for restraint of dangerous animals, e.g. a bull or steer amok in public places. **Warning**: etorphine can be life-threatening to the operator if absorbed by any route. Extreme care should be taken. Before any use of Immobilon™ the appropriate dose of the antagonist Revivon™ (contained in the same pack) should be drawn up first into a second syringe, which should then be kept close at hand for immediate intravenous use in the event of an accident. A second person should always be instructed clearly beforehand what action should be taken with the reversing agent, which should then be injected *before* calling medical assistance.

Indications

Use with a dart gun (i.e. intramuscular injection) for restraint of dangerous and uncontrollable cattle.

Dosage:

0.5–1 ml Immobilon™ per 50 kg bodyweight i.m. by dart syringe. Cattle become recumbent some minutes later, and remain immobile for about 45 minutes. Generalised muscle tremors and poor muscle relaxation are usually apparent.

To reverse the drug an equal volume of Revivon™ (diprenorphine HC1) should be injected i.v. Recovery generally occurs with minimal disturbance and noise. A second half dose of Revivon™ may be given s.c. after the initial i.v. dose if required.

Operator warning (from UK data sheet of LA Immobilon™/Revivon™)

To avoid accidental self-injection two sterile needles should be used, one to fill the syringe, the second to inject the patient. After the calculated dose has been withdrawn from the vial, the syringe should be removed from the needle. The syringe should be connected to a second needle immediately before delivery. Both needles should be discarded into a closed labelled container. Operator should wear rubber gloves and should not pressurise vial contents. Veterinarian should fully brief assistant on accident procedure and administration of the reversing agent (LA Revivon™) should any Immobilon™ be inadvertently absorbed through skin, mucous membranes (mouth, eyes) or through injection.

Immobilon is highly toxic, causing dizziness, nausea, pinpoint pupils, rapidly followed by respiratory depression, hypotension, cyanosis, loss of consciousness and cardiac arrest.

The reader should consult specialised textbooks (see Further Reading section, pp. 259–60) for further details of bovine GA.

1.10 Shock

A state in which there is inadequate perfusion of tissues. Shock lesions result from:

- failure of homeostatic mechanisms to maintain adequate perfusion
- homeostatic mechanisms themselves reduce perfusion by eliciting excessive production of various vasoactive hormones, amides, peptides and kinins

Shock may eventually become refractory to treatment. Inadequate perfusion is due to failure of blood flow, not of blood pressure. Changes are due to hypoxia and accumulated metabolites from defective perfusion. Basic pathology: necrosis of cells and tissue, haemorrhages and fibrin thrombi in venous circulation (Shwartzman). Almost every organ displays lesions.

Shock in bovine practice may be due to various states, for example:

- hypovolaemic shock as a result of massive haemorrhage, namely reduction of circulating blood volume to less than 80% (reduction to less than 65% in critical)
- dehydration, e.g. 10–12% is severe, and over 15% is critical
- burns, e.g. third degree burns over more than 25% of body surface
- infection – septic shock, especially gram-negative bacteria liberating endotoxins (e.g. generalised Shwartzman reaction)
- peripheral vascular disease with gangrene
- spinal anaesthesia (cranial or epidural, see Section 1.8, pp. 27–29)
- acute haemolytic conditions

A fall in blood pressure as a result of shock due to severe systemic blood loss triggers off a sequence of events in which the animal attempts to maintain an adequate blood supply to the brain and coronary vessels, but which may compromise other tissues (see Figure 1.16). Prompt fluid therapy is often the most important corrective measure in such cattle.

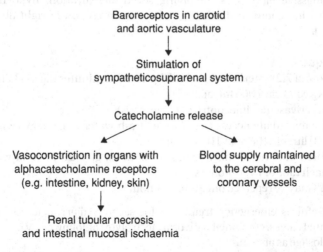

Baroreceptors in carotid
and aortic vasculature

↓

Stimulation of
sympatheticosuprarenal system

↓

Catecholamine release

Vasoconstriction in organs with
alphacatecholamine receptors
(e.g. intestine, kidney, skin)

Blood supply maintained
to the cerebral and
coronary vessels

↓

Renal tubular necrosis
and intestinal mucosal ischaemia

Figure 1.16 Summary of some reactions following severe blood loss and shock.

1.11 Fluid therapy

Introduction
Correction of fluid and electrolyte deficits may be critical in severe shock and blood loss, in conditions such as right abomasal volvulus (see Section 3.7, p. 110) and in severe, protracted toxic cases of bovine dystocia. A water deficit can result from anorexia, dysphagia, diarrhoea and hyperosmolality.

Fluids

Dehydration is expressed as a percentage of total reduction of body fluids and is estimated as follows:

- persistent skin fold for > 3 seconds
- prolonged capillary refill (> 4 seconds)
- sunken eyeball or enophthalmos e.g. 7 mm recession indicates about 12% dehydration

Volume of fluid required for replacement is calculated very simply: litres required = bodyweight in kg × % dehydration. For example, a 500 kg cow with 10% dehydration requires 50 litres of fluid to cover her deficit.

Intravenous catheters are usually placed into the jugular vein following skin preparation (Cathlon® IV, Johnson & Johnson, Intracath®, Becton Dickinson 16 G or 19 G for calves, 10 G or 12 G for rapid infusion in cows).

Hypertonic saline (HS) (see Table 1.11)
Hypertonic saline (HS) is a major advance in fluid therapy for haemorrhagic shock (massive blood loss) involving severe dehydration, hypovolaemic shock and in endotoxic shock (e.g. following correction of right abomasal volvulus).

Technique
- i.v. dose of 7.2% sterile saline, 4 ml/kg over five minutes (i.e. 2–3 litres to a 600 kg cow) via 10 G (Intracath®)
- avoid perivascular injection (tissue necrosis)
- ensure immediate access to unlimited fresh water (most cows will drink 20–40 litres in the next 10 minutes)
- if patient does not drink within five minutes, give 20 litres of water by stomach tube or i.v. isotonic saline
- i.v. HS may be repeated once after 24 hours

HS is useful as emergency treatment for severely diarrhoeic and (> 8%) dehydrated calves, combined with oral electrolytes or followed by i.v. isotonic saline (dosage as above).

Electrolytes

Introduction

Ideally, the solution is selected after determining the individual animal's needs by laboratory evaluation. However on the farm this is not practical. In general cattle have rather consistent acid base and electrolyte abnormalities associated with surgical disease. Dehydrated cattle are twice as likely to have metabolic alkalosis as metabolic acidosis. Alkalosis is treated by giving a solution rich in chloride and potassium. Given adequate circulatory volume and electrolytes, the kidneys can usually correct the alkalosis.

Oral rehydration can be achieved rapidly (e.g. 20 litres of dextrose and/or saline in less than three minutes) using a stomach pump attached to an oesophageal tube, which is protected from damage by the cow's teeth by a straight outer sleeve, one end of which has nose tongs attached for insertion into the nostrils. Dehydration is easily corrected in adult cattle if combined with i.v. therapy (see below) or sometimes alone to prevent, for example, borderline ketosis.

Replacement rules (see Table 1.11)

- K is reduced in abomasal volvulus (see Section 3.7, p. 111) and is associated with metabolic alkalosis: it should be replaced with KCl
- K is also reduced in diarrhoeic conditions: replace with K_2CO_3
- Na is reduced in abomasal torsion, and involves metabolic acidosis; replace with 0.9% NaCl or KCl

Table 1.11 Composition of six fluids given as replacement therapy to cattle.

	Electrolyte concentration (mEq/litre)						
	Na^+	K^+	Ca^{++}	NH_4^-	Cl^-	HCO_3^-	Lactate$^-$
Normal plasma	140	4	5	0	103	25	5
0.9% NaCl	154	0	0	0	154	0	0
Ringer solution	145	4	6	0	155	0	0
Lactated Ringer	130	4	3	0	109	0	28
Hypertonic saline (7.2%)	120	17	7[0]	0	144	0	0
Ammonium KCl solution*	0	75	0	75	150	0	0

* Whitelock, R.H., et al. (1976) Proceedings of the International Conference of Production Diseases of Farm Animals, 3 edn. Wageningen, The Netherlands, pp. 67–9
[0] if $CaCl_2$

Calculation of electrolyte quantities

(a) Calculate total extracellular fluid (ECF) volume: ECF (litres) = body-weight in kg × 0.3. For example, a 500 kg cow has 150 litres ECF

(b) Deficit of Na^+ and/or Cl^- is estimated by laboratory biochemistry; the difference between normal and calculated values is the deficit per litre

(c) The deficit of K^+ is unreliable if calculated from plasma K, but twice this calculated deficit may be safely administered if:

● renal function is satisfactory

● K^+ is given as K_2CO_3 or KCl well diluted in other fluids, at 10–20 mEq/litre and infusion rate per hour does not exceed 100 mEq K^+ in adult (500 kg) cow. K^+ may often be easily given in drinking water later (about 40 mEq/litre as K_2CO_3 or KCl).

1.12 Anti-microbial chemotherapy

Introduction

Anti-microbial drugs are no substitute for sound and aseptic surgical technique in sterile aseptic procedures, neither can they be expected to control deep-seated necrotic and purulent foci. These drugs should be considered as adjuncts to the natural defence mechanisms of the host. The primary aim is to improve these mechanisms by proper preparation of the surgical field, surgeon and the instruments, appropriate débridement, excision of necrotic tissue, drainage and lavage, together with the prompt re-establishment of the nutritional fluid, electrolyte and acid-base balance of the patient.

One example is septic arthritis where joint lavage with saline is indicated (see Section 7.27, p. 257) and may sometimes be replaced by more radical open joint surgery, supported by systemic and local anti-microbial chemotherapy. Antibiotic prophylaxis is not required during clean surgical procedures in cattle (e.g. LDA abomasopexy, entropion surgery).

Prophylactic antibiotic therapy is however indicated in extensive abdominal surgery, open fracture repair and non-sterile invasive procedures. This therapy should start before the surgical intervention, the therapeutic concentration should already be adequate at the start of surgery and the intravenous route is preferable. The dose rates of prophylactic and therapeutic antimicrobials are similar.

In contaminated sites, such as caesarean hysterotomy following prolonged unsuccessful vaginal manipulation and a dead fetus, rectal tears requiring extensive suturing, or in surgical sepsis, an adequate tissue concentration of antibiotic should be rapidly established and therapy should continue for at least three to five days after surgery. Initial anti-microbial drug selection is usually arbitrary (broad spectrum) and may be altered following results of sensitivity testing.

Table 1.12 Some guidelines for the antimicrobial sensitivity of certain drugs against common bovine pathogens (see footnote).

Organism	Antimicrobial drug First choice	Alternative choice (s)
Arcanobacterium pyogenes	Amoxicillin (c)	Penicillin G (c)
Staphylococcus aureus		
nonpenicillinase	Penicillin G (c)	amoxy/clav (c)
penicillinase	Oxacillin (c)	amoxy/clav (c)
Clostridium spp.	Penicillin G (c)	Tetracycline (Cl. tetani) (s)
Escherichia coli	Marbofloxacin (c)	Ampicillin (c)
Fusobacterium	Ceftiofur	Penicillin G (c) Tetracycline (s)
Enterobacteriaceae	Aminoglycosides Marbofloxacin (c)	Carbenicillin (c)
Klebsiella	Marbofloxacin (c)	Cephalosporin (c)
Pasteurella	Ceftiofur, Enrofloxacin[‡]	Tetracycline[†] (s) Trimethoprim + sulpha (s&c)
Proteus mirabilis	Ampicillin (c)	Marbofloxacin (c)
other *Proteus*	Marbofloxacin (c)	Carbenicillin (c)
Salmonella	Trimethoprim + sulpha (s&c)	Ampicillin (c)
Streptococcus	Penicillin (c)	amoxy/clav (c)

Note: enormous variations exist between different laboratories and countries, also antibiotic legislation is very variable, therefore obtain advice from nearest veterinary laboratory!
(c) = bactericidal; (s) = bacteriostatic; (s/c) = bactericidal in high concentrations only
[†] widespread resistance of *Pasteurella* spp. to tetracycline is recognised; alternative drugs are sulfachlorpyridazine or erythromycin
[‡] use in USA restricted to beef cattle

The most common bovine pathogens and their sensitivity are shown in Table 1.12. The sensitivity may be variable depending on the area and country.

Reasons for a failure of sensitivity testing are listed in Table 1.13. A failure of response to anti-microbial therapy can be due to a variety of other reasons (see Table 1.14).

The problem of milk withdrawal times in lactating dairy cattle must be kept in mind (see Table 1.15). Currently ceftiofur HCL (e.g. Excenel RTU® sterile suspension, [Pfizer]) is a very popular systemic antimicrobial as it has a nil milk withdrawal time.

Table 1.13   Failure of sensitivity testing (susceptibility) to predict outcome of therapy: some possible factors.

Impaired absorption
Accelerated elimination
Adverse drug interaction(s)
Inadequate penetration/drainage
Reduced phagocytosis
Drug antagonism
Superinfection
Impaired normal host defences
Underlying disease
Genotypic or phenotypic drug resistance
Tolerance

Table 1.14   Failure of response to antimicrobial therapy: list of possible factors.

Absence of concurrent surgical/mechanical measures, e.g. drainage
Inappropriate drug selection or dosage
Sensitivity testing: organism resistant *in vitro*
Predisposing and management factors remaining uncorrected
Misdiagnosis, as condition not of bacterial origin
Impaired immune function
Fluid electrolyte, acid-base imbalance, nutritional defects
Inflammation, with release of mediators, cellular breakdown products, oedema, tissue
   destruction, coagulation, impaired perfusion and penetration
Poor management of mixed infections involving anaerobes
Toxin elaboration before antibacterial concentration is obtained at infection site
Drug resistance, therapeutic, prophylactic, growth promotion use
Compliance
Underlying disease or concurrent medication
Adverse reactions: toxicity

In summary, in cattle anti-microbial selection should be based on the organism's sensitivity, predicted drug tissue levels, confidence in drug safety and cost, and approval of extra-label use in each country.

Post-surgical analgesia may be improved by flunixin meglumine (Finadyne®, [Schering-Plough] Ketoprofen® [Rhone Merieux]), or meloxicam (Metacam®, Boehringer Ingelheim). Flunixin meglumine, when used at label dose, incurs ten days of meat withholding and three days' milk withholding in the United States (respectively 5 and 1 days in UK).

Table 1.15 Effective therapeutic period and withdrawal times of chemotherapeutic agents in UK and USA (2004/2005). Since drugs are given in various forms and strengths, milk discard times and withdrawal times will vary accordingly: *drug labels should always be checked*!

Drug	Effective therapeutic period (days)	Milk discard UK	Milk discard USA	Slaughter (meat) UK	Slaughter (meat) USA
Ceftiofur Na (Naxcel®)	1	0	0	0	0
Ceftiofur HCl (Excenel®)	1	0	0	8	0
Trimethoprim/Sulphadiazine	1	6.5	2.5	34	5
Oxytetracycline 100	1	4	4	21	7–22
Oxytetracycline LA	4	7	4	14	28
Procaine penicillin G	1	2–5	2	3–4	10
Procaine penicillin G + streptomycin	1	2.5	2	23	30
Ampicillin	1	1–7	2	18–60	6
Erythromycin	1	2	3	7	14
Amoxicillin	1	1–7	NP	18–42	25
Framycetin	1	2.5	NA	49	28–38
Cefalexin sodium	1	0	4	19	4
Florfenicol (Nuflor®)	2	NP	NP	30–44	28–38
Clav. acid/amoxicillin (Synulox®)	1	2.5	—	42	—
Enrofloxacin (Baytril®)	1	3.5	NP	14	28

NA = not available, NP = not permitted
British readers are referred to the current data sheets and the current NOAH Compendium.
US readers should refer to the Center for Veterinary Medicine, see Appendix 3 (p. 267)

1.13 Wound treatment

Successful surgical treatment of wounds depends on:

- thorough débridement
- meticulous haemostasis
- elimination of dead space
- proper use of instruments
- judicious insertion of drains
- proper placement of sutures

Since the healing process is basically similar in all species (see Figure 1.17), these points all apply to cattle. Bovine wounds fortunately heal without production of exuberant granulation tissue which is commonly seen in the horse.

Débridement is essential, especially when the wound (e.g. teat) is to be sutured and in areas when gross contamination is commonplace.

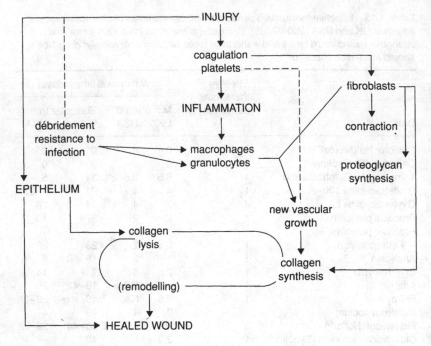

Figure 1.17   Basic process of wound healing.

Haemostasis prevents haematoma formation in dead space which would potentially offer an ideal culture medium for bacterial growth.

Dead space may be packed with sterile gauze swabs for 24–48 hours to prevent haematoma formation (see Section 2.7, pp. 69–70).

Drains are rarely indicated in cattle except for certain long bone fractures, the thorax or subcutaneous or deep infected wounds (e.g. laparotomy incisions) where:

- irrigation is required several times daily
- the outflow of infected material may be ensured without the need regularly to reopen the lower end of the incision

Sutures in wounds:

- do not suture infected wounds

Irrigation of wounds:

- large volume of clean non-sterile fluid (e.g. mains water) is more valuable than small volume of sterile physiological saline
- ensure all pockets of deeper wounds are reached by irrigation fluids
- judicious use of 3% hydrogen peroxide, or 1% chlorhexidine solution speeds removal of pus and tissue debris
- development of dead space may be prevented by judicious closed active drainage (suction drainage, Redon type drain)

Skin sutures: single or interrupted mattress sutures of sheathed polyamide polymer multifilamentous material (e.g. Vetafil®, Supramid® [Braun]), monofilament nylon or polypropylene (see Table 1.5, p. 9)

Deep sutures in infected wounds: PGA, PDS

Drains:

- Penrose
- sialastic
- polypropylene, flexible and thin-walled with multiple openings in deeper tissues

1.14 Cryotherapy

Introduction
Advantages of this technique include:

- frequently faster than knife surgery
- little or no haemorrhage
- relative absence of post-operative complications
- phenomenon of cryo-immunity may delay or prevent neoplastic regrowth

Disadvantages are few:

- objectionable odour resulting from tissue necrosis
- risk of uncontrolled freeze resulting in destruction of vital tissues

Materials, termed cryogens, are:

- liquid nitrogen (N) (boiling point $-196°C$)
- nitrous oxide (N_2O)($-89.5°C$)
- carbon dioxide (CO_2)($-35.5°C$)

Equipment
Equipment may be small and readily portable (special vacuum flask), or can be rather large and heavy, e.g. Frigitronics CE-8. Operator should wear

disposable protective plastic gloves and avoid any possibility of cryogen contacting the skin of involved personnel. General anaesthesia may be necessary for delicate cryotherapy, since the affected area must be kept immobile during treatment.

Technique

- wash and dry area and apply a little paraffin jelly or vaseline (e.g. KY® jelly) for improved initial adhesion
- if spray is to be used, mask off surrounding area with piece of plastic sheet or with thick layer of vaseline
- select suitable probe head (e.g. flat, 10 mm or 20 mm diameter) or spray attachment (2.36–1.25 metric needle, depending on desirability of coarse or fine spray)
- if necessary attach flexible extension piece to keep apparatus vertical and a short distance from operating site
- if available, and working near vital structures, insert thermocouples: drop of reading to −20°C is critical and indicates need to arrest cryotherapy at once
- in absence of thermocouples and in most situations in cattle, digital assessment of size and position of iceball is quite reliable
- produce rapid freeze and permit slow thaw cycle; two cycles necessary for N, three for N_2O or CO_2
- assess extent of iceball by digital palpation. Probe is removed after natural thaw, or after activating automatic defrosting device
- do not repeat freeze until area is completely thawed. Effectiveness of procedure depends on sequence of rapid freeze-slow thaw cycles
- warn owner or stockperson to anticipate tissue necrosis and slough in seven–ten days, leaving a healthy granulating surface, which should be kept clean as epithelialisation proceeds from periphery inwards

Discussion

Factors affecting degree of cryonecrosis include:

- probe temperature – liquid nitrogen is capable of freezing any tissue in the body
- size of probe tip – the greater its diameter the greater the volume of frozen tissue
- size of spray orifice – the larger the orifice, the greater the concentration of cryogen applied to lesion, resulting in very rapid freeze and larger volume of frozen tissue. With liquid nitrogen, spray orifice penetrates much deeper and faster than probe tip, though latter is more precise
- duration of freeze – at temperatures below −20°C for 1 minute or more virtually all living tissue undergoes cryonecrosis. The longer the freeze, the larger the iceball.

1.15 Coccygeal venepuncture

Indications
Collection of venous samples (volume up to 10 ml) with minimal restraint and little or no assistance. Obvious advantages over collection from jugular or subcutaneous abdominal (milk) vein (latter not recommended). Minimal risk of infection and sporadic haematoma formation insignificant, so tail paralysis is virtually unknown.

Technique
Collect into evacuated blood collection tubes containing edetic acid (EDTA), heparin etc., or without coagulant (Vacutainer® [Becton Dickinson, Rutherford, NJ]) via 0.9 metric 4 cm needle which is screwed into plastic holder into which collection tube is inserted. Alternatively collect via 0.8 metric 2 cm needle into polypropylene syringe (5–10 ml) with negative pressure.

- restrain head in stall by chain or halter, or in squeeze chute or head gate (manual restraint rarely required)
- grasp tail in middle third and slowly elevate to almost vertical position ('tail jack' Figure 1.18)

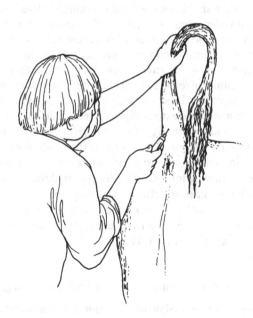

Figure 1.18 Method of restraint for obtaining blood samples from coccygeal vein.

- cleanse tail site of gross faecal contamination with paper towel or cotton wool
- with free hand locate palpable vein in midline, just caudal to insertion of skin folds of tail at level of coccygeal (Co) vertebrae 6–7
- insert needle just cranial to bony protuberance of haemal process in midline to depth of about 8–12 mm (in Vacutainer® system, insert needle into tube), and withdraw slightly until bloodflow starts
- if initially unsuccessful, reduce tension of tail slightly and continue at same site, otherwise attempt at Co 5–6
- do not massage puncture site after venepuncture

Other reports claim that sites of Co 3–5 are preferable, but anatomical studies show the vein lies to the right of midline in the ventral sulcus of the vertebral body at the more cranial site.

Insignificant haematoma develops in a small number of cases, but disappears in a few days. Procedure does not cause thrombophlebitis or total occlusion of vein, and repeat samples are easily obtained some days or weeks later.

1.16 Hereditary defects

Introduction
Until the 1960s congenital defects in cattle were thought to be largely heritable. There has been a slight but perceptible change in this attitude of veterinarians, cattle breeders and geneticists. 'Congenital' is not synonymous with 'heritable' or 'genetic'. There remains a great paucity of information. A limited number of conditions can be corrected surgically, and where it is likely that the condition is inherited, steps should be taken (e.g. castration, sterilisation, or crushing of teats) to avoid breeding from such stock.

Incidence of congenital defects in cattle is 0.2–3%, with 40–50% born dead. Most defects are visible externally. Congenital defects reduce the value of affected calves, and frequently of their normal relatives too. Economic losses are particularly severe when congenital losses are combined in a syndrome involving embryonic and fetal mortality. Such losses are often increased by longer calving intervals resulting from dystocia and subsequent infertility. Breeding programme changes subsequent to such incidents may require the introduction of less popular and profitable stock.

Close collaboration between veterinarians, farmer and geneticist is essential. Good breeding records are a vital tool.

Examples
Examples of the more common defects of each body system are:

- skeletal – single and isolated defects include spinal abnormalities such as scoliosis, kyphosis, tibial hemimelia, polydactyly, syndactyly

- systemic skeletal defects – chondrodysplasia (dwarfism), osteopetrosis
- joint defects – arthrogryposis and congenital muscle contracture ('ankylosis'), hip dysplasia, bilateral femorotibial osteoarthritis
- muscular – arthrogryposis, congenital flexed pastern and/or fetlocks, muscular hypertrophy
- spastic paresis
- CNS – internal hydrocephalus, spina bifida, Arnold Chiari malformation (herniation of cerebellar tissue through *foramen magnum* into cranial cervical spinal canal) cerebellar hypoplasia, cerebellar ataxia, spastic paresis, spastic syndrome
- skin – epitheliogenesis imperfecta, entropion
- cardiovascular – ventricular septal defect, patent *ductus arteriosus*
- digestive – atresia of ileum, colon, rectum and anus
- hernias – umbilical, scrotal/inguinal, schistosomus reflexus
- reproductive – testicular hypoplasia, intersex (hermaphrodite and freemartin), ovarian hypoplasia, rectovaginal constriction (Jerseys) and prolonged gestation

Many of the above musculoskeletal defects (e.g. muscular hypertrophy or double muscling in the Belgian Blue) can give rise to dystocia.

Surgical correction of several of these defects is considered elsewhere: umbilical hernia (see Section 3.13, p. 122), rectal and anal atresia (see Section 3.18, p. 133), and spastic paresis (see Section 7.21, p. 246).

CHAPTER 2

Head and neck surgery

2.1 Disbudding and dehorning

Indications
- improve stock management
- prevent potential aggressive behaviour towards other members of herd and stock personnel
- reduce traumatic damage to such persons and other individuals and stock, especially udder and skin injury resulting in eventual lowered hide value

Selection of technique
In the UK all calves over one week old may only be disbudded or dehorned under anaesthesia or analgesia (Animal Anaesthetics Act 1964). In some other countries (e.g. Switzerland), regardless of age, anaesthesia is mandatory. Under proposed animal welfare guidelines, it is suggested that dehorning (not disbudding) may ultimately be outlawed. The veterinarian should strive, under Herd Health Plans, to convince farmers to disbud at an early age.

Very young calves (< 1 week old) may be disbudded by application of a local caustic compound (NaOH, KOH, collodion). Wear protective gloves. Clip hair from horn buttons. Protect surrounding skin with petrolatum, and apply thin film of paste. Confine calves for 30 minutes. Use of caustic preparations may be forbidden in some countries (e.g. Switzerland).

The ideal age for disbudding is one to two weeks old, when horn buds project 5–10 mm, are easily palpable, and a disbudding iron can be used alone (see Figure 2.1a,c). Haemorrhage is nil.

From about one to four months (horn length 3–5 cm) a Barnes dehorning gouge (see Figure 2.1b,d), Roberts dehorning trephine, or double action hoofshears may be applied, followed by a disbudding iron for haemostasis. Alternatively the Danish debudding gouge is available. The bud and peripheral

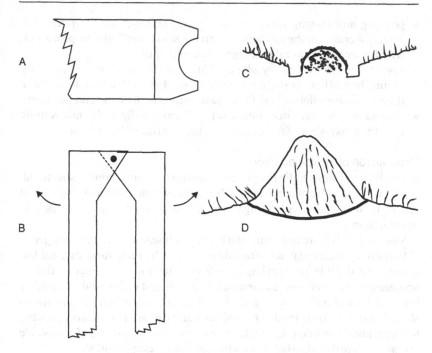

Figure 2.1 Two disbudding and dehorning instruments (not to scale).
A. head of electrical or gas-powered calf disbudding iron; B. Head of Barnes dehorner;
C. and D. are cross-sections of effect in C burning a circular trough around bud; in
D. blades cut away horn and rim of adjacent skin.

skin may be removed by forceps and scissors following trephination. Older
animals (older calves, yearlings, adults) are dehorned either by embryotomy
(Gigli) wire, Barnes gouge, dehorning (butcher's) saw or dehorning shears.

Analgesia: block of cornual nerve (see Section 1.8, pp. 18–20).

Calves may be adequately handled in pens. Stock over nine months (e.g.
200 kg) are preferably put through a crush/chute, a group of 10–20 being
blocked and marked in sequence before carrying out the dehorning.

Some breeds have a significant proportion of polled stock (e.g. Hereford) or
are all naturally polled (e.g. Aberdeen Angus).

Technique of disbudding
- restrain calf with hindquarters in corner and head held by thumb and
  fingers placed between and below jaws, assistant leaning against shoulder
  region
- place hot (electrical or gas-powered) disbudding iron on bud and rotate
  several times, angling the instrument so that the edge burns the skin
  around the periphery of the bud to include adequate germinal epithelium
  (see Figure 2.1c)

- pressing and moving head laterally, scoop and flick off the horn bud, leaving a crater, in the middle of which is a small cartilaginous protusion, which may be left since it is not germinal epithelium
- operate on older calves by placing blades of Barnes dehorner precisely around base of horn bud and removing small (3–5 mm) strip of skin at same time as bud is guillotined off. Effect haemostasis with hot disbudding iron
- alternatively remove horns as short as 5 cm rapidly with embryotomy wire (more physical effort but minimal haemorrhage due to heat)

Comparison of instrumentation

In yearling and adult cattle the preferred method is embryotomy (obstetrical, Gigli) wire, disadvantages being the considerable physical effort and relatively slow speed. Advantages include neat appearance and lack of haemorrhage.

Saw method is more unsightly and control of haemorrhage takes longer.

Dehorning shears (e.g. Keystone dehorner) is the most rapid method but causes considerable haemorrhage and has a major disadvantage in that, if analgesia is absent or poor, sudden violent movement of the head (avoided by firmly anchored halter!) during closure of the guillotine blades can cause a shear fracture of the frontal bone and secondary wound problems including frontal sinusitis. In addition the shears method raises questions of acceptable animal welfare if analgesia is not confirmed before its application.

Dehorning of cattle without demonstrable analgesia is an unethical and unprofessional act.

Technique of dehorning

- sedation occasionally indicated
- cornual nerve block (see Section 1.8, p. 19). In adult cattle infiltrate further anaesthetic solution at caudal border of horn base
- wait five to ten minutes
- check with needle that skin adjacent to horn is painless
- obtain adequate restraint of head in gate of crush and position head straight forward so that considerable weight can be exerted on embryotomy wire during sawing movement (see Figure 2.2). Likewise, when using saw, ensure that operator's position is optimal
- first cut is made with wire or saw on lateral aspect
- place wire and saw so that instrument passes through skin about 1 cm from skin-horn junction
- ensure that direction is correct, especially with saw, since change of direction brings greater difficulties in moving blades
- ensure that blade or wire emerges dorsally through skin lateral to midline of poll. In Friesian/Holstein cows width of skin left in midline should be 5–8 cm
- avoid interrupting sawing movement in middle of dehorning process

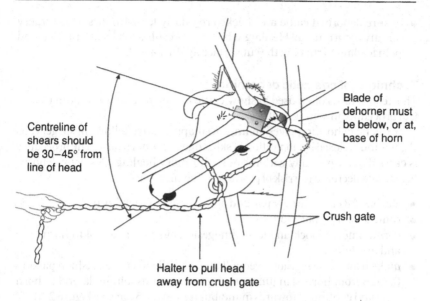

Centreline of
shears should
be 30–45° from
line of head

Blade of
dehorner must
be below, or at,
base of horn

Crush gate

Halter to pull head
away from crush gate

Figure 2.2 Position of cow's head and of dehorning shears (Keystone) or saw.
Note that (a) haltered head is pulled forwards away from crush gate, and to side;
(b) cutting angle should be 30–45°; (c) blade or wire is placed onto skin of
horn-skin junction.

Relatively narrow diameter horns (< 5 cm) may be removed using long-handled dehorning gouge (Barnes pattern). This instrument may also be useful in removing additional protruding lips of horn where the initial procedure has been too conservative.

Haemostasis

- torsion or torsion/traction on the 2–3 major vessels in the medial aspect (ventral crescent) of the peripheral skin; they are easily identified and picked up by artery haemostatic forceps, six to eight turns are optimal
- rubber tourniquet or string around the two horn bases (such as rubber bands made from cross-sections of car inner tubes or baling twine) applied in pattern to exert pressure on dorsal horn border as well
- alternatively push wooden toothpick into bone canal from which considerable blood can spurt (remove toothpick the next day)
- cautery, e.g. hot iron, electrocautery, is often disappointingly ineffective
- liberal use of bacteriostatic (e.g. non-sterile furazolidone or sulphanilamide) or haemostatic powder (Fe salts, tannic acid, alum)

- ensure dehorned cattle are checked regularly for 24 hours after surgery for any recurrence of bleeding which may result from local irritation and pain leading to rubbing the cut surface against a wall

Technique of cosmetic dehorning

This technique is often used in show cattle in North America. It is an unethical procedure in some countries.

Cosmetic dehorning gives an improved appearance following surgery, as the wound is closed by apposition of skin edges over horn base. The procedure is carried out aseptically with the aim of primary healing. Cosmetic dehorning should decrease the risk of post-operative sinusitis.

- clip band 8 cm wide over poll and around base of each horn
- routine skin preparation
- cornual nerve block and local analgesic infiltration caudal to horn base and in midline
- make transverse incision over poll and laterally in curved fashion passing 0.5 cm from horn-skin junction, the two wounds joining lateral to horn base and continued towards mandibular joint for 5 cm (see Figure 2.3)
- undermine skin peripherally from incision far enough to avoid skin damage when horn is removed by saw or Barnes dehorning gouge
- remove more horn if necessary (sterile bone chisel and hammer, Barnes gouge) until cut is exactly flush with frontal bone
- clean surface with sterile swabs and effect haemostasis
- undermine skin further to enable edges to be apposed across bone surface without excessive tension, then check cosmetic appearance
- appose edges with interrupted sutures of monofilamentous polypropylene
- clean surface of all blood and debris, and apply antibiotic powder
- remove sutures in 14 days

Complications and discussion

Complications of disbudding and dehorning include:

- side-effects caused by inadvertent i.v. injection of analgesic solution in young calves (excessive salivation, mild ataxia, temporary collapse)
- failure to remove the horn bud completely in calves (inadequate depth of cauterising activity) results in regrowth or 'scurs'
- in older cattle frontal sinusitis (pneumatisation of the horn starts at eight to nine months) and empyema caused by entry of infection and fly strike in summer and autumn. Therefore avoid dehorning in the major fly season (e.g. in UK May to late September). Also avoid feeding hay or straw from overhead racks to reduce risk of frontal sinusitis.

Crude surgical technique results in prolonged local irritation and increased tendency for cut surface to be rubbed against dirty surfaces (e.g. soil, bedding,

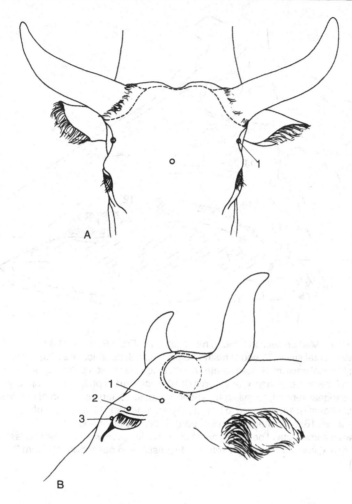

Figure 2.3 Incision and nerve supply for cosmetic dehorning. (A) Rostral view;
(B) lateral view.
1. zygomatico-temporal nerve; 2. frontal nerve; 3. infratrochlear nerve; --- skin
incision.

walls). Most infected wounds can be cleaned easily, but infection extending
into the frontal sinus can cause chronic discharge of pus (often *A. pyogenes*) to
pass into the maxillary region, sometimes with systemic illness (e.g. pyrexia,
anorexia, loss of condition, head tilt, localised swelling and pain). Drainage
by sinus trephination may then be indicated (see Section 2.2 below).

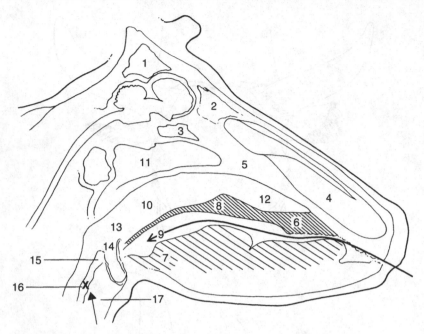

Figure 2.4 Median section through head, left half. (From Pavaux, 1983.)
1. caudal frontal sinus; 2. medial rostral frontal sinus; 3. sphenoidal sinus; 4. nasal cavity; 5. nasal septum; 6. hard palate; 7. root of tongue; 8. soft palate; 9. *isthmus faucium* (oral part of pharynx, oropharynx); 10. nasal part of pharynx (nasopharynx); 11. pharyngeal septum; 12. nasopharyngeal meatus; 13. laryngeal part of pharynx (laryngopharynx); 14. entrance to larynx (laryngeal aditus); 15. vestibule of oesophagus; 16. oesophagus (cervical part); 17. cavity of larynx.
X shows common site of oesophageal obstruction; long arrow shows hand passed into pharynx, and short arrow the retrograde pressure on oesophagus. (From Pavaux; 1983.)

2.2 Trephination of frontal sinus (for empyema)

Indication
Frontal sinusitis with considerable volume of pus occupying the multi-loculated structure and with chronic discharge through the horn base.

Anatomy (Figures 2.4 and 2.5)
The frontal sinus is comprised of several compartments (see Figures 2.4 and 2.5). The large caudal frontal sinus is completely divided by an oblique partition into a rostromedial and a caudolateral portion. The former has a narrow nasofrontal opening and a post-orbital diverticulum. The latter has

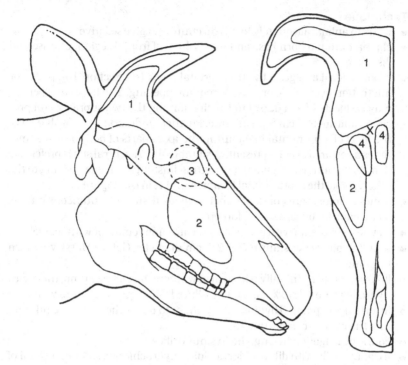

Figure 2.5 Diagram of longitudinal and rostral sections through skull to show extent of sinuses.
1. frontal sinus; 2. maxillary sinus; 3. position of orbit; 4. rostral compartments of frontal sinus; X trephine sites for empyema of frontal sinus. (Modified from Dyce & Wensing, 1971.)

the cornual diverticulum and nuchal diverticulum which ends by also excavating the parietal, occipital and temporal bones. Two or three small chambers lie level with the rostral part of the orbit.

The borders of the frontal sinus are from the rostral part of the orbit to a transverse line drawn through the midline of the orbit, laterally to the frontal crest, and caudally to the nuchal crest (poll). A midline septum separates the two frontal sinuses. The normal small communication of the frontal sinus with the ethmoid sinus and the nasal cavity is usually occluded due to thickening of the mucosa and purulent discharge.

For clinical signs of frontal sinus empyema see section on complications of dehorning (see Section 2.1, p. 58). Some cases result from horn fracture, usually a direct result of uncontrolled movement of the head (poor anaesthesia). Sinusitis is often confined initially to caudal part of sinus.

Technique

- restrain animal adequately in crush/chute and give sedative
- clip hair around horn base and over whole of frontal region, cleanse and disinfect
- produce local analgesia by supra-orbital block (see Section 1.8, p. 20) or infiltration over site of proposed trephine opening. The trephine opening may be located 5 cm dorsal to the line joining the two supra-orbital processes and about 5 cm from midline. Further landmark: 2–3 cm abaxial at the level of a horizontal line joining the axial parts of both orbits. Sometimes a soft area of bone presents a suitable site. A ventral site is preferable if the horn sinus is still patent, permitting flushing from one opening to the other. Avoid the supra-orbital foramen and vein (see Figure 1.4)
- remove circular area of skin, subcutaneous tissue and cutaneous muscle 3 cm diameter by scalpel and forceps
- elevate periosteum with periosteal elevator and remove it with scalpel
- trephine bone over sinus using 2.5 cm diameter Galt or Horsley pattern trephine
- flush sinus cavity initially with warm water using enema pump, then with hydrogen peroxide (3%, i.e. 10 vol, diluted with equal volume of water)
- insert enema pump (Higginson's syringe) to direct the irrigating mixture into the various compartments
- continue irrigation through horn sinus orifice
- irrigate finally with dilute chlorhexidine hydrochloride solution (10 ml of 5% solution made up to 1 litre with water), flushing from top to bottom
- pick up any major bleeding points with artery forceps and maintain trephine opening patent for daily flushing by stock person
- avoid feeding hay/straw from overhead rack

In chronic cases repeated lavage or a permanent through-and-through lavage system may be needed.

The wound usually heals in three to four weeks. Parenteral medication (five to ten days with broad spectrum antibiotics) is indicated in animals with systemic signs and in all longstanding and severe cases. As trephine opening closes over, irrigation should be continued with a flexible polypropylene or PVC catheter attached to the syringe. It is a good idea to suture the catheter in place. Prognosis is favourable (acute cases) to guarded (chronic cases). Infection rarely extends to the opposite side of the skull or to the CNS.

Discussion

In consideration of the possible and safe sites for trephination, note that the site for euthanasia using a captive bolt gun is midline at the junction of diagonal lines joining the medial canthus of the orbit to the ventral border of the opposite horn base (see Figure 2.3a).

2.3 Entropion

Incidence and signs

- low incidence, more common in some beef breeds
- involves and lower lid more frequently than upper lid
- often bilateral to varying extent
- occasionally congenital, usually acquired
- signs include mild blepharospasm, conjunctivitis, keratitis, and corneal ulceration if not corrected early
- conservative non-surgical treatment often successful e.g. manual eversion, injection of saline into lid, horizontal mattress tacking suture in eyelid

Indication

- correction of congenital or acquired inversion of upper or lower lid

Technique (Hotz-Celsus procedure)

- estimate length and width of skin to be resected by pinching to produce approximate skin fold to correct inversion of lid margin
- linear s.c. infiltration of anaesthetic solution parallel and 2 mm distant to lid margin
- scalpel incision to remove ridge of skin previously measured (see Figure 2.6)
- close wound margin with single continuous or mattress absorbable suture e.g. PDS (avoiding need for later removal)
- complications unlikely, though under-correction may necessitate second surgery

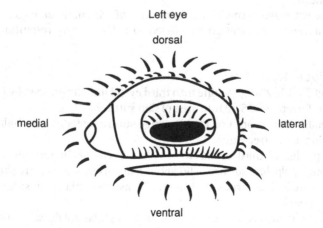

Left eye

dorsal

medial

lateral

ventral

Figure 2.6 Entropion correction involving lower lid of left eye with skin incision 2 mm below lid margin.

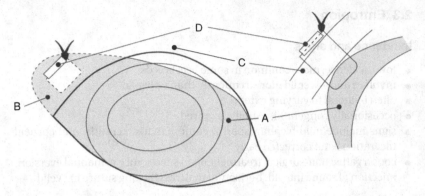

Figure 2.7   Third eyelid flap in right eye. Shaded area is third eyelid A. sutured into dorsolateral fornix; B. by suture through skin; C. supported by 1.5 cm long plastic stent D. Note that suture does not penetrate full depth of third eyelid, therefore does not contact corneal surface.

2.4 Third eyelid flap

A suture placed in the third eyelid (nictitating membrane) is passed through the dorsal lateral conjunctival fornix to emerge through the skin. When tightened the third eyelid is drawn across the corneal surface.

Indications

Cases of extensive corneal ulceration and of traumatic damage, often in which antibiotic medication has failed to achieve early resolution of the lesion.

Technique (Figure 2.7)

- inject 2 ml 1–2% lignocaine into third eyelid initially grasped by fine Allis tissue forceps, and 5 ml into area of skin sutures
- thread PGA (Dexon®) or PDS 0 gauge suture material onto half-curved cutting needle (see Figure 1.2 (5))
- grasp edge of third eyelid with Allis forceps again and place suture through palpebral surface of lid about 5 mm from edge. Suture should not penetrate bulbar surface of third eyelid (as this could result subsequently in corneal abrasion)
- now insert each end of suture in turn through lateral dorsal conjunctival fornix to emerge through skin about 2–3 cm above lateral commissure of eyelids

- insert 1 cm polypropylene stent onto suture over skin, and tie in 'quick release' fashion with sufficient tension for third eyelid to cover entire visible surface of cornea, including the lesion
- inspect eyelid suture daily (stockperson), apply any local medication and perhaps slacken off suture to inspect cornea for assessment of healing process
- leave suture in place for two to three weeks, then remove with scissors

Complications and their reasons
- early tearing out of suture from third eyelid, resulting from insufficient 'bite'
- failure to pull flap sufficiently laterally due to incorrect placement of conjunctival and skin suture, usually too medial in position
- pulling out of sutures through skin due to absence of stent
- mechanical irritation of corneal surface from suture material (suture perforated entire depth of third eyelid, or was too slack, failing to pull third eyelid completely across corneal surface)

Discussion
No comparative studies are available on the success of this simple and common technique. Results are generally good as bovine cornea has great powers of healing.

2.5 Neoplasia of eyelids

Introduction
Neoplasms of the upper and lower lids and nictitating membrane (third eyelid) include squamous cell carcinoma (SCC) or 'cancer eye', and rarely other tumours such as papillomata, and fibrosarcoma. SCC is most significant in terms not only of incidence but also of economic importance and prognosis. SCC occurs more frequently on the globe (65%) than upper and lower lids (30%) or third eyelid (5%), is very invasive locally, and may metastasise to the local lymph nodes (parotid, atlantal or retropharyngeal and the anterior cervical chain).

Clinical signs
SCC is largely confined to Hereford and Simmental breeds and their crosses, where the non-pigmented area is liable to develop neoplastic lesions under the influence of ultraviolet radiation from sunlight. Affected cattle are usually four to nine years old. About 85% of cattle with SCC lack pigment in the affected area.

The lesion is often an obvious proliferative irregular mass which may ulcerate through the skin to cause moderate distress and blepharospasm.

Early lesions appear either as rice-grain-like plaques on the sclera or corneal surface, or as small firm nodules in the dermis. This precursor of a greyish-white plaque at the nasal and temporal limbus develops into a papilloma and carcinoma *in situ*. Lid lesions often start as a dirty brown, horn-like keratomata.

Treatment

Treatment is indicated in early lesions without evidence of secondary spread to adjacent structures (e.g. bone) or metastases to the drainage lymph nodes.

Several techniques are available and include:

(a) excisional surgery
(b) cryotherapy
(c) hyperthermia
(d) radiotherapy (rare)
(e) immunotherapy (rare)
(f) combinations of a+b, a+d or c+e

Excisional surgery of third eyelid

- in standing or recumbent animal induce analgesia by local infiltration (5 ml of 2% lignocaine) of base of eyelid after instilling topical anaesthetic solution (e.g. 0.5% proparacaine) into conjunctival sac
- draw third eyelid out by traction with forceps
- excise eyelid deep to cartilage with curved scissors
- control haemorrhage with adrenaline-soaked swab, or cryotherapy

Cryotherapy

Cryotherapy (see Section 1.14, p. 49) is particularly advantageous since the technique avoids haemorrhage and is simple and relatively fast. The small liquid nitrogen flask (Nitrospray® [Arnolds]) is adequate for lesions up to 5 cm diameter and 1 cm deep.

- protect eye from inadvertent freezing by inserting 'Styrofoam' strips or acrylic between lid and corneal surface. Apply water-soluble lubricants or vaseline to skin of surrounding healthy area
- clip and wash affected area and put on disposable rubber gloves
- freeze the area twice (liquid nitrogen) or three times (nitrous oxide, carbon dioxide) initially using a spray tip
- include at least 5 mm width border of clinically healthy tissue
- evert tissue lying close to cornea by grasping with towel clips or Allis tissue forceps, before applying probe head which is designed to deal with lesions of the third eyelid
- use thermocouples if available, inserting points 5 mm from margin of lesion and stopping freeze when they indicate a temperature drop below −20°C

Advantages of cryotherapy over knife surgery in treatment of SCC are:

- simple, cheap and rapid method
- good post-operative analgesia
- minimal pre-operative preparation and usually no post-operative medication necessary
- procedure may be repeated if there are multiple lesions
- no bleeding

Disadvantages of cryotherapy are:

- lesions > 2.5 cm diameter require relatively prolonged application of probe head for complete iceball formation
- lesions exceeding 5 cm must be treated in two stages, alternatively an initial surgical debulking procedure
- initial instrumentation cost is high, but treatment cost per lesion is then low

Other techniques

- excisional surgery: often indicated in large lesions to reduce size ('debulk') prior to cryotherapy
- radiofrequency hyperthermia: application of heat (50°C for 30 seconds) to various surface points of tumour and surrounding skin using probe head. Penetration is limited to 0.5–1 cm, therefore inappropriate for large masses
- radiotherapy: radon and gold seed implants have both been successfully used in valuable cattle. Penetration is again only 0.5–1 cm
- immunotherapy: local infiltration of mycobacterial cell wall fraction immunostimulant (Regressin® [Ragland], USDA-approved drug for immunotherapy). Dose rate is 0.5 ml for each centimetre of tumour diameter, i.e. 5 cm diameter mass is given 2.5 ml. It is claimed that untreated sites often undergo spontaneous regression
- Prognosis: recurrence possible

2.6 Ocular foreign body

Introduction
Foreign bodies such as particles of chaff, burrs and thorns may lodge on the corneal surface, particularly in lateral or medial canthus, and provoke a reactive keratoconjunctivitis. Signs are obvious in recent cases with epiphora, ptosis, blepharospasm and discomfort. Chronic cases show corneal scarring and pigmented keratitis. Such material may often be removed without local analgesia. Suitable topical analgesics include amethocaine (e.g. Minims® Amethocaine HCL, [Smith & Nephew Pharmaceuticals]), xylocaine (4% eyedrops – Astra®), or Proparacaine (Ophthaine®, Ophthetic®).

Technique
- hold head firmly and tilted in good light so that material is, as far as practical, in midfield of orbital fissure
- spray sterile saline through 22 gauge needle hub tangentially at foreign body to dislodge it
- if unsuccessful then attempt dislodgement and removal with fine dissecting forceps or with fine flat surface such as blunt surface of large scalpel blade
- assess superficial corneal damage subsequent to removal, following instillation of one to two drops of fluorescein stain (Minims® Fluorescein sodium 1% or 2% [Smith & Nephew Pharmaceuticals])
- insert local broad spectrum antibiotic (e.g. cloxacillin, Orbenin®, [Beecham]) four times daily for three days after removal. Ointments are more suitable than drops. Topical 1% atropine b.i.d. or to effect to maintain pupil dilatation. Corticosteroids may be contra-indicated as they hamper repair of any residual ulcer.

2.7 Enucleation of eyeball

Indications
- intra-ocular neoplasia and gross damage to bulb, usually with severe primary or secondary infection, e.g. infectious bovine keratoconjunctivitis (*Moraxella bovis* ± *Neisseria* spp.) associated with trauma or rupture of globe, resulting in anterior staphyloma or panophthalmitis, and risk of ascending infection up the optic stalk.

Enucleation is rarely indicated in cattle. Cosmetically satisfactory appearance is not so important as in equines and small animals.

Technique of transpalpebral enucleation (exenteration)
- anaesthesia: preferably GA, but alternatively standing or recumbent under xylazine sedation and retrobulbar block (see Section 1.8, p. 21), or ophthalmic nerve analgesia and local infiltration of lower lid and medial canthus
- clip and cleanse peri-orbital area
- place continuous suture through upper and lower lids
- perform lateral canthotomy (2 cm) to aid exposure
- using traction with towel clips or Allis tissue forceps, make circumferential incision 1 cm from skin – conjunctival junction, or as appropriate depending on the distribution of non-viable or neoplastic skin (see Figure 2.8)
- continue towards orbital ridge down to, but not through, conjunctiva
- exerting some traction on eye muscles, dissect the extra-ocular muscles bluntly with Mayo scissors from lateral and medial canthus. Avoid excessive traction on optic nerve.

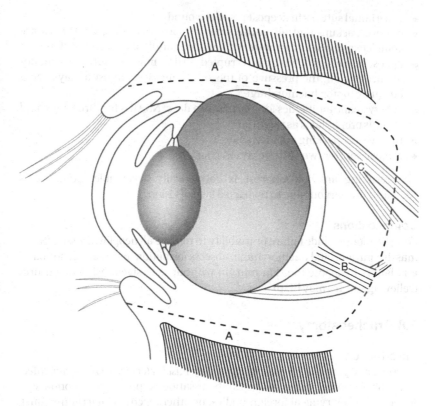

Figure 2.8 Exenteration of eye (longitudinal diagrammatic section). Dotted line (A) starts in the lids, passes through the peri-orbital structures and results in removal of globe, all orbital contents, eyelid margin and conjunctiva. B. optic nerve and vessels; C. muscles. Shaded areas above and below are frontal and zygomatic bones.

- grasp eyeball and use further traction to dissect it free from surrounding retrobulbar tissue (excluding conjunctival sac) and optic nerve
- leave the maximal amount of healthy retrobulbar tissue
- clamp ophthalmic vessels, optic nerve and retractor bulbi muscle with slightly curved, long-handled artery forceps (Roberts 23 cm, or Kelly 25 cm)
- ligate vessels with 7 metric chromic catgut
- remove third eyelid and Harderian gland
- check site for complete removal of all neoplastic or infected tissue
- meticulous haemostasis during enucleation is time-consuming and in most cases not necessary
- pack the orbital space for a few minutes with sterile gauze while subcutaneous layer of simple interrupted sutures of chromic catgut is inserted, or insert absorbable gelatinespmges

- place initial sutures in deepest point of wound
- remove packing and all gauze swabs before subcutaneous tissues are completely closed and irrigate with aqueous antibiotic solution (20 ml)
- appose skin edges of lids by interrupted vertical mattress sutures of monofilament nylon, the pressure of the suture incision almost always being adequate to stop haemorrhage
- give systemic antibiotics for five to seven days, NSAIDs for three days, and tetanus prophylaxis as required
- remove any packing after two days
- remove sutures two to three weeks later

The resulting ankyloblepharon is cosmetically acceptable. Some cows become more nervous due to restricted field of vision.

Complications
Complications include failure or inability to remove all neoplastic tissue (SCC), massive intra-orbital haemorrhage, abscess formation, excessive dead space, and failure to appose the skin margin without excessive tension on sutures (relieving sutures may help).

2.8 Tracheostomy

Introduction
Necrotic and purulent laryngitis (caused by *Fusobacterium necrophorum* infection and *Arcanobacterium pyogenes* abscessation respectively) secondary to intra- or retro-laryngeal foreign bodies, or other mechanical irritants (dust, repeated coughing due to *Haemophilus somnus* and other pathogens).

Indications for tracheostomy rarely involve pharyngolaryngeal neoplasia, retropharyngeal abscessation, foreign bodies in upper respiratory tract, or persistent laryngospasm. Surgical conditions of head involving haemorrhage and potential aspiration of blood and infected tissue should be managed with an endotracheal tube in position. Tube should only be removed after return of cough and swallow reflexes.

Clinical signs
Signs indicative of need for tracheostomy, which is often an emergency procedure, include progressive dyspnoea, stridor, and mild cyanosis. Some animals have fetid breath (*F. necrophorum*), and pharyngeal lesions which can be both seen and palpated. In all cases a mouth gag should be inserted and a long-bladed laryngoscope or endoscope used to aid examination of the affected area.

Anatomy
Tracheal rings are readily appreciated on deep palpation of upper part of neck. Diameter is narrow compared with equine trachea. Depth is slightly

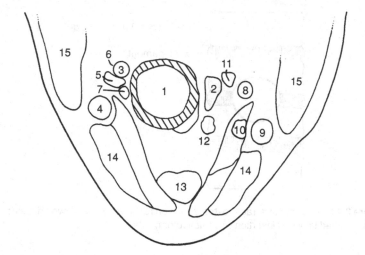

Figure 2.9 Cross-section of neck at level of fifth cervical vertebra, ventral part, looking caudally.
1. trachea; 2. oesophagus; 3. right common carotid artery; 4. right external jugular vein; 5. right internal jugular vein; 6. right vagosympathetic trunk; 7. right recurrent laryngeal nerve; 8. left common carotid artery; 9. left external jugular vein; 10. left internal jugular vein; 11. left vagosympathetic trunk; 12. left recurrent laryngeal nerve; 13. sternohyoid and sternothyroid muscles; 14. sternocephalic muscle; 15. brachiocephalic muscle. (From Pavaux, 1983.)

greater than width. Trachea is related at junction of upper and middle thirds of neck to oesophagus on left side, and to carotid sheath, enclosing common carotid artery, vagosympathetic trunk and internal jugular vein on the right and to a lesser extent on the left. The trachea is approached through the two bellies of the bulky sternomandibular muscles and the finer sternothyrohyoid muscles, which are fine muscular bands on the ventral tracheal surface (see Figure 2.9 which is a cross-section somewhat distal to preferred tracheostomy site).

Technique
- perform surgery on standing, haltered animal (in crush/chute) under local infiltration of analgesic solution (2% lignocaine with adrenaline)
- premedicate difficult animals with xylazine, but avoid premedication in animals with signs of severe cardiovascular and respiratory dysfunction
- maintain head and neck in extension
- identify midline in upper half of neck at level of tracheal rings 4–6
- clip and disinfect skin over this area and make longitudinal incision 6 cm long through skin and subcutis directly over the tensed trachea
- separate the paired sternomandibular muscles in midline by blunt dissection, followed by sternothyrohyoid muscles

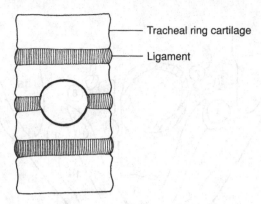

Tracheal ring cartilage

Ligament

Figure 2.10 Diagram of a tracheostomy incision to show portion of two adjacent rings resected to permit insertion of a tracheotomy tube.

- insert self-retaining wound retractor (West or Gossett model)
- incise tracheal annular ligament and grasp adjacent tracheal ring with forceps
- resect two half-moon shaped segments of adjacent tracheal rings corresponding to size of the tracheal tube (see Figure 2.10). This form of tracheal incision maintains the lumen of the adjacent trachea
- insert tracheal tube. Various models are available. A small size (25 mm diameter) steel equine tube may be used in emergencies. In an immature animal (calf) the maximum diameter may be 13 mm; these are commercially available (39 FG). Some tubes are up to 14 mm diameter (Portex Blue Line®) and have external tapes for fixation
- anchor tube to skin at a minimum of two points to prevent rotation

In **emergency situation**, with no other equipment available, insert a ⁺50–70 cm length of vinyl stomach tubing, 16 mm or 19 mm (external diameter) and suture in place around tracheotomy wound and also tape over parotid region.

In cattle any tracheotomy tube requires frequent (minimum twice daily) cleaning of both tracheal lumen and external surface. The relative quantity of debris and inflammatory discharge is greater than in horses.

- remove tube after alleviation of primary condition, which may require systemic antibiotherapy alone, or combined surgery (drainage of laryngeal abscess in calves) and antibiotherapy
- do not suture the wound
- avoid hay dust in the immediate environment to reduce likelihood of iatrogenic bronchopneumonia

Sometimes a major complication is the extension of granulation tissue from the wound edge to partially occlude the tracheal lumen. Resect such proliferative tissue by electrocautery.

Prognosis remains guarded in all cases.

2.9 Oesophageal obstruction

Introduction

Oesophageal obstruction is usually due to round or irregular pieces of food material, e.g. potato, turnip or sugar beet, rarely to sugar beet pulp (cf. horse). It can usually be relieved by medical means (e.g. tranquillizers such as phenothiazine derivatives, relaxants) and manual retrograde manipulation.

Site of obstruction is usually the proximal cervical oesophagus, often in the first 20 cm (see Figure 2.4, (x)) and rarely the distal cervical or thoracic oesophagus.

Distal thoracic oesophageal obstruction is sometimes seen in calves due to 'broken' stomach feeders following oral rehydration therapy. Rarely oesophageal obstruction results from external compression (thymic lymphosarcoma, mediastinal lymphadenopathy) and neurogenic dysfunction (rabies).

Oesophageal obstruction is rarely life-threatening as long as care is taken to control development of rumenal tympany. Insert temporary rumenal canula. Oesophagotomy should be a last resort procedure.

Oesophagotomy is only practical in proximal two-thirds of the cervical part, where organ is relatively accessible, lying in deep fascia to left of the trachea and overlaid by the left jugular vein and the carotid sheath enclosing the carotid and vagosympathetic trunk.

Oesophagotomy (for anatomy see Figure 2.9)

- identify site of obstruction and, if not palpable, ascertain by gently passing stomach tube
- delay radical surgery a minimum of 24 hours, pending medical relief (e.g. xylazine)
- perform surgery under GA or with sedated animal in right lateral recumbency
- infiltrate local anaesthetic solution after routine skin preparation
- carry out surgery with strict aseptic precautions
- keep tissues tense and surgical field convex, elevated by underlying pad or by sterile assistant, and attempt again to move FB retrograde into pharynx
- incise skin adequate length (twice the length of foreign body) and bluntly dissect down to oesophageal wall
- carefully reflect jugular and carotid trunk dorsally
- incise thin oesophageal wall longitudinally and carefully remove obstruction, using gauze swabs to avoid contamination of surgical field by saliva and food debris

- close oesophageal wall (unless necrotic) with interrupted absorbable sutures attached to swaged-on curved round-bodied needle
- place sutures 5 mm apart through mucosa and muscularis
- oversew muscularis in second layer of simple continuous PGA sutures, including fascia for increased strength
- irrigate area well with sterile saline before routine skin closure
- insert Penrose drain along external oesophageal wall to emerge at ventral (caudal) commissure of skin wound in cases where contamination is thought likely to lead to infection and secondary healing
- remove drain after 48 hours
- do not suture oesophagus in cases of full depth mural necrosis, but leave as open fistula

Though lying adjacent to oesophagus, it should be easy to avoid damage to the common carotid artery (dorsolateral) and jugular vein (ventrolateral). Cattle with reversible neurogenic oesophageal dysfunction may be supported by alimentation through a rumen fistula.

Distal oesophageal obstruction ('broken' stomach feeders, see above) is treated by removal via rumenotomy incision.

Prognosis
It is difficult to ensure the primary healing of oesophageal incision, but chances are increased by keeping animal on fluids for two days, followed by three days of mash and short-cut fodder.

CHAPTER 3

Abdominal surgery

3.1 Topography

Topography of the forestomachs and abomasum (see Figure 3.1) is incorporated in descriptions of approach (e.g. left flank laparotomy, traumatic reticulitis). The complex topography of the intestinal tract is considered in this introduction.

The intestinal tract

The small intestine includes the duodenum (cranial, descending and ascending parts), jejunum, and ileum. The large intestine is comprised of the caecum, ascending colon (proximal loop, spiral loop [centripetal and centrifugal coils], distal loop), transverse colon, descending colon and rectum.

Position and course

The muscular pylorus lies fairly fixed in position supported by the origin of the lesser omentum dorsally and the greater omentum ventrally, and situated level with the costochondral junction of ribs 9 and 10 on the right side (see Figures 3.2, 3.3 and 3.24). The cranial duodenal loop passes craniodorsal,

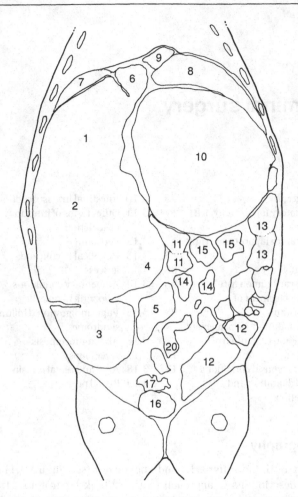

Figure 3.1 Horizontal section of trunk at mid-height of thorax and thighs, looking ventrally.
1–5. rumen: 1. atrium (cranial sac); 2. dorsal sac; 3. caudodorsal blind sac; 4. ventral sac; 5. caudoventral blind sac; 6. reticulum; 7. spleen; 8. liver; 9. caudal vena cava; 10. omasum; 11. jejunum; 12. caecum; 13–15. ascending colon: 13. proximal loop; 14. spiral loop; 15. distal loop; 16. urinary bladder; 17. uterine horns. (From Pavaux, 1983.)

initially freely mobile, but with the next portion firmly adherent to the visceral hepatic surface. It curves in an S-shaped manner near the bile and pancreatic duct openings, and becomes the descending loop, which is suspended dorsally by the mesoduodenum, and the loop passes caudally in the dorsal and right lateral part of the abdominal cavity (see Figure 3.2). Superficial and deep parts of the greater omentum attach to the ventral surface of the descending loop of the duodenum.

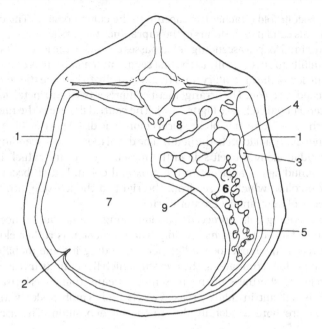

Figure 3.2 Distribution of greater omentum, viewed diagrammatically through a vertical section of abdomen, about lumbar vertebra 3.
1. parietal peritoneum; 2. insertion into left longitudinal groove of the rumen of the superficial layer of the greater omentum; 3. duodenum; 4. mesoduodenum (cranially the lesser omentum); 5. deep and superficial layers of greater omentum; 6. intestinal mass in supra-epiploic recess; 7. rumen; 8. left kidney; 9. deep layer of greater omentum inserting onto right longitudinal groove of rumen. (Modified from Dyce & Wensing, 1971.)

The duodenum turns craniad at the caudal flexure, where it is attached to the descending colon by the duodenocolic ligament, and becomes the ascending loop to pass cranial to the left side of the mesenteric root. It turns to the right side of the root to become the jejunum.

The jejunum, 35–50 m long, comprises a mass of tight coils at the edge of the mesentery. The greatest intestinal mass is formed by these heaped coils of jejunum. The mesentery of the proximal and middle sections is short, that of the distal part and that attached to the ileum are longer, forming a mobile section which lies caudal to the supra-omental recess. The ileum comprises a convoluted proximal segment and a distal straight part. The junction of jejunum and ileum is the point where the cranial mesenteric artery ends, and the cranial limit of the ileocaecal fold. The ileum is attached to the caecum ventrally, the orifice lying obliquely on the ventral surface of the caecum, and readily identified in adulthood due to the fat pad overlying it.

The caecum is a mobile sac, with the blind end directed caudally. Cranially the caecum is continuous with the proximal loop of the ascending colon. The short caecocolic fold attaches the caecum to the colon dorsally. The caecum often extends caudal to the limits of the supraomental bursa.

The proximal loop of ascending colon passes cranial to the level of T12 then turns caudally to pass dorsally to the first segment. It again turns craniad, but now to the left of the mesentery, and then ventrally to become the spiral loop of the ascending colon. The arrangement comprises two centripetal, followed by two centrifugal coils (see Figure 3.3). The central flexure is the mid-point and the change in direction of the spiral colon. The distal portion of the spiral colon is normally adjacent to the ileum. The distal loop of the ascending colon passes caudad along the left side of the mesentery, around which it turns to run craniad again, adjacent to the proximal colon. It then becomes the transverse colon, which passes from the right to the left side, around the cranial edge of the cranial mesenteric artery.

The descending colon proceeds caudad along the dorsal surface of the abdomen, attached by the mesocolon. The mesocolon is rather elongated at the level of the duodenocolic ligament, affording it some mobility. The descending colon terminates in the rectum, which lies entirely intrapelvic.

The relative shortness of the mesentery means that exteriorisation of intestine is difficult in many areas. Vessels and lymph nodes within the mesentery are hard to identify due to the fat deposition. The ascending

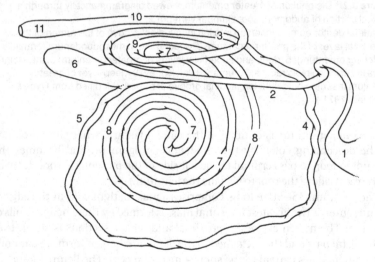

Figure 3.3 Diagrammatic representation of small and large intestine, viewed from right side.
1. pylorus; 2. descending limb of duodenum; 3. ascending limb of duodenum;
4. proximal jejunum; 5. distal jejunum and ileum; 6. caecum; 7. proximal loop and centripetal gyri of colon; 8. centrifugal gyri of colon; 9. ascending terminal colon;
10. descending colon; 11. rectum. Length (in adult) of small intestine is 40 m, that of the large intestine is 10 m.

duodenum, proximal and distal loops of ascending colon, and the cranial portion of the descending colon lie close to one another due to the near-fusion of their mesenteries. The cranial mesenteric vessels supply the small and large intestine, except for parts of the duodenum and colon.

The greater omentum passes from its origin on the duodenum, pylorus and greater curvature of the abomasum, encircles the intestinal mass, and inserts on the left longitudinal groove of the rumen (superficial part), while the deep part passes similarly ventral and to the left, to attach to the right longitudinal groove of the rumen. These two parts are fused caudally forming the caudal fold. The lesser omentum extends from the oesophagus along the reticular groove and omasal base to attach to the lesser curvature of the abomasum, and covers most of the parietal surface of the omasum.

Abdominal viscera (see also Fig. 3.7)

Viscera which contact left abdominal wall (see Figures 3.1, 3.2, 3.4 and 3.5):

- cranially and ventrally: reticulum
- laterally ribs 10–12 dorsally, ribs 7–8 ventrally: spleen
- laterally: rumen covered ventrally by greater omentum from left longitudinal groove
- laterally and (sublumbar) dorsally: perirenal fat
- ventrally and caudally: sometimes coils of jejunum and ileum

Viscera which contact right abdominal wall:

- cranially and ventrally: reticulum and abomasum
- laterally and cranially (ribs 7–12): liver
- laterally (rib 7 ventrally, rib 12 dorsally); descending loop of duodenum and small intestine covered by greater omentum

Viscera which do not normally contact body wall:

- omasum at level of ribs 8–11, lying ventrally to right of midline
- caecum and ascending colon (caudal mid-abdomen), transverse and descending colon
- left kidney (level with vertebrae 2–4), and right kidney (thoracic vertebra 13–lumbar 2)
- uterus and ovaries: uterus in advanced pregnancy (gestation month seven) may contact lower left and/or right flank

3.2 Exploratory laparotomy (celiotomy), left flank

Indications

Specific indications are suspected left displaced abomasum (LDA) (see Section 3.6), rumenotomy, traumatic reticulitis (see Section 3.4), or caesarean

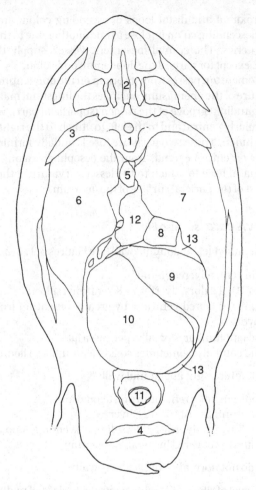

Figure 3.4 Cross-section of thorax through body of seventh thoracic vertebra, looking cranially.
1. body of seventh thoracic vertebra; 2. spinous process of sixth thoracic vertebra; 3. seventh rib; 4. sternum; 5. thoracic duct and aorta; 6. left lung; 7. right lung; 8. caudal vena cava; 9. liver; 10. reticulum; 11. apex of heart; 12. accessory lobe of right lung; 13. central tendon and sternal part of diaphragm. (From Pavaux, 1983.)

section (see Section 4.1). LDA is evident on opening into peritoneal cavity. Traumatic reticulitis may be suspected on exploration of area between cranial aspect of ruminoreticulum and the diaphragm-body wall area. In positive cases specific surgical correction is performed.

Indication is often not clearcut. Some cattle show persistent abdominal pain apparently localised to ruminal area. Left flank exploratory laparotomy

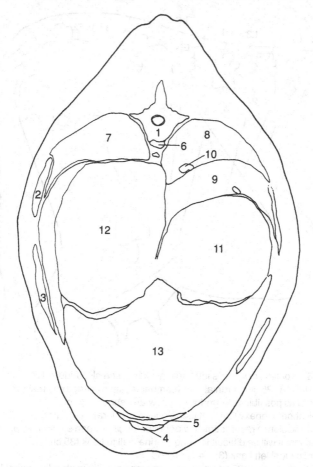

Figure 3.5 Cross-section of trunk through body of ninth thoracic vertebra, looking cranially.
1. body of ninth thoracic vertebra and head of ninth rib; 2. eighth rib; 3. seventh rib; 4. xiphoid process of sternum; 5. sternal part; 6. thoracic aorta (thoracic duct, to right, and left azygos vein to left, coursing along it dorsolaterally); 7. left lung (caudal lobe); 8. right lung (caudal lobe); 9. liver; 10. caudal vena cava; 11. omasum; 12. atrium (cranial sac) of rumen; 13. reticulum. (From Pavaux, 1983.)

is rarely as useful or as practical as right flank approach and is not recommended if a small or large intestinal surgical disorder is suspected.

Laparoscopic surgery is being developed in cattle for abdominal exploration and treatment of LDA but is currently mostly confined to referral clinics.

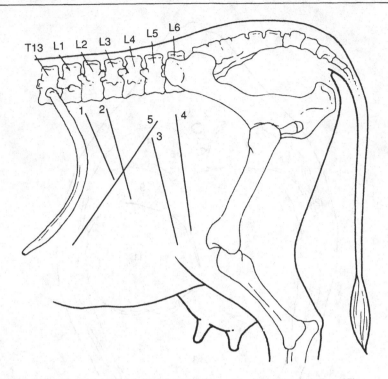

Figure 3.6   Position of various left flank incisions (see also Figure 1.7, p. 25).
1. paracostal (18–25 cm), cranial in sublumbar fossa: rumenotomy (essential to be as far cranial as possible in large-framed cow and short surgeon);
2. left flank abomasopexy (Utrecht technique) or exploratory laparotomy (25 cm);
3. low flank incision in recumbent cow or heifer for caesarean section, where it is anticipated that it will be difficult to bring uterine wall to flank (35 cm);
4. standard caudal left flank (35–40 cm) and
5. oblique flank incision (35–40 cm) for caesarean section in standing animal.

Technique
- paravertebral analgesia (T13, L1 and L2, see Section 1.8, pp. 22–26) or local infiltration (see Section 1.8, pp. 26–27)
- clip, scrub and surgically prepare a wide area of left flank including at least 30 cm around proposed incision site (see Figure 3.6)
- drape with sterile cloths or rubber drape with appropriate window
- make paracostal incision 15 cm long about 5 cm behind last rib, starting 10 cm below lumbar transverse processes
- incise skin in single movement and continue scalpel incision through sub-cutaneous fat and fascia to expose abdominal wall musculature

- insert blade of straight scissors at angle of 45° to surface and into external oblique abdominal muscle, which is separated by blunt dissection
- make 7 cm long scalpel incision through internal oblique muscle to expose underlying transverse fascia
- make small incision with scissors through this fascia to reveal parietal peritoneum beneath a variable amount of loose fat
- pick up parietal peritoneum with rat-tooth forceps and make small vertical incision with scissors
- extend incision through internal oblique, transverse fascia and peritoneum with scissors to correspond to length and direction of skin incision. Air rushes audibly into abdominal cavity at this point creating pneumoperitoneum, and contact surface of ruminal wall (unless adhesed) drops away as abdominal wall moves laterally. (Occasionally some pneumoperitoneum is present before surgery, e.g. in traumatic reticulitis.)

Left side of abdominal cavity and part of right side may now be explored (see Figure 3.7).

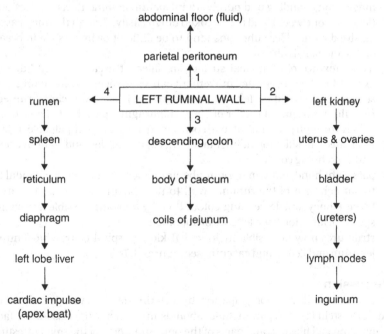

Figure 3.7 Flow diagram of left flank exploratory examination. As in right flank approach (see Figure 3.8) entire accessible part of abdominal cavity should be rapidly checked in any abdominal disease. Start from left ruminal wall with palpation of parietal peritoneum (1), then caudal abdomen (2) and the right side structures (3), before concentrating on left flank and left cranial and ventral regions (4).

Visible features

- check volume and colour of peritoneal fluid; normal colour is pale yellow. A slight pink tinge may be due to contamination of some blood from incision site. Presence of any floccules, usually purulent, is abnormal and indicates an infective focus in the visceral or parietal peritoneum. Possibly also an associated objectionable odour.
- run fingers over surface of both parietal and ruminal (visceral) peritoneum adjacent to incision: surface should be smooth. Irregularities may be in form of discrete adhesions or generalised lesion ('sandpaper-like') consistent with chronic peritonitis.

Palpable features

- introduce the right hand and arm to make systematic examination of the abdominal cavity (see Figure 3.7)
- pass right hand ventrally to check for possible LDA, and also cranially for adhesions between reticulum and diaphragm or liver, or (rarely) between rumen and abdominal wall, suggestive of traumatic reticulitis
- presence of abdominal adhesions may be of recent origin and significant, or may be longstanding and purely an incidental finding. Recent adhesions (less than one week) tend to be broken down easily, though this may cause localised pain. Older adhesions tend to be difficult or impossible to break down and pain is absent
- assess texture of peritoneal surface in different areas at early stage of exploration before repeated movement causes iatrogenic roughening
- structures palpated on left side (see Figure 3.1) should include: rumen, reticulum, spleen, left border of liver, diaphragm, apical beat of heart, left kidney through perirenal fat, path of ureters (normally non-palpable unless thickened), bladder including bladder neck, uterus, left and right ovaries, and descending colon
- pass right hand and arm to right abdominal wall by directing it caudal to the attachment of the ruminal wall to the abdominal roof, and ventral to left kidney and descending colon, thereby avoiding possible iatrogenic spread of infection from left side of abdomen
- structures now accessible include: left kidney, spiral colon, duodenum, jejunum and ileum, and caecum (see Figures 3.1–3.3).

Discussion

Structures too distant for palpation by veterinarian of average stature in adult Holstein Friesian cow include: abomasum, much of the visceral surface of liver and gall bladder, and parts of the omasum, some of the small intestine (jejunal loops) and large intestine (colonic coils).

3.3 Exploratory laparotomy, right flank

Right laparotomy site is corresponding position to that of left paralumbar fossa (incision 2 in Figure 3.6). Ensure that ventral commissure of incision is in upper half of flank, otherwise spontaneous prolapse of greater omentum and some small intestinal (jejunal) coils is almost inevitable. Take special care in peritoneal incision as descending duodenum is immediately below!

Visible features

Note greater omentum below incision, with descending duodunum passing caudally in the omentum.

Palpable features

- pass left hand and arm ventrally to palpate abomasum, note some mobility is possible and abomasum may be grasped and pulled upwards towards incision
- appreciate cranially visceral surface of liver (note any rounded edges, abscesses or surface irregularity) with dependent gall bladder (normal size up to $10 \times 6 \times 4$ cm), and insert hand between liver and diaphragm to palpate cranial hepatic surface, e.g. discrete abscessation
- pass hand along lateral body wall with palm outwards and ventrally locate reticulum (note any adhesions, or foreign bodies) beyond abomasum and greater omentum
- check contact area of reticulum with diaphragm (possible adhesions)
- note mesoduodenum is dorsal to duodenum, and deep to this area is the perirenal fat (right kidney)
- palpate, caudal to right kidney, the right surface of left kidney, both structures being slightly to right of midline due to pressure from rumen. Right kidney is dorsal to cranial part of descending duodenum, to right of mesoduodenum. Left kidney lies adjacent to middle part of descending duodenum entirely within the supraomental recess
- pass hand caudal to caudal edge of greater omentum which runs approximately midway between last rib and *tuber coxae*
- palpate structures in this space, which include numerous coils of jejunum and ileum, as well as spiral colon, caecum, which is very variable in size, and dorsally ascending colon and descending colon (see Figure 3.3)
- some intestine which may be exteriorised for examination includes much of jejunum (except cranially), apex and body of caecum, and more ventral loops of ascending spiral colon
- note, suspended from midline (palpable but cannot be exteriorised), descending colon and part of ascending colon, passing into pelvic cavity together with bladder, uterus and ovaries

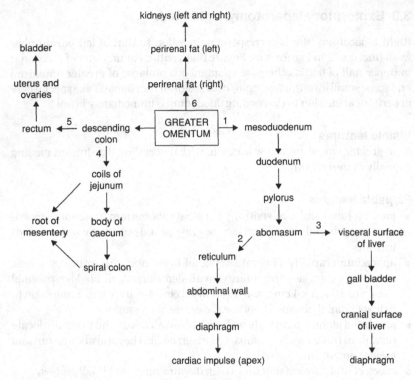

Figure 3.8 Flow diagram of right flank exploratory laparotomy. Entire accessible abdominal cavity should be checked in any case of suspected abdominal disease. In a case of LDA the abomasum is not found on right side (step 1), but against left abdominal wall. Nevertheless steps 2 and 3 should be followed to rule out co-existing traumatic reticulitis or liver abscessation. In suspect cases of small or large intestinal disease or displacement, step 4 should be followed, but exploration of remainder of abdominal cavity should be carried out at a later stage.

Closure of flank laparotomy incision

- close the incision in three layers (see Figure 3.9a)
- appose peritoneum and transverse fascia with continuous suture of 4 metric PDS on 3/8 circle round-bodied needle
- commence suture at ventral commissure and tie off dorsally
- close external and internal oblique abdominal muscles separately or together with similar single layer
- appose skin with Ford interlocking suture of monofilament nylon or Supramid® inserted with cutting-edged semi-curved needle. A relatively fine needle about 5 cm long requires less effort to insert through 5–7 mm thickness of skin than a larger needle

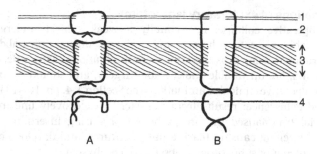

Figure 3.9 Transverse section through flank (diagrammatic) showing two methods of closing laparotomy wounds. (A) Recommended three layer closure; (B) single layer figure-of-eight closure.
1. peritoneum; 2. transverse fascia/muscle, 3. internal and external oblique muscles; 4. skin.

- close ventral 5 cm with interrupted sutures which may be removed later for drainage of any wound infection
- note that in all three layers sutures should be just tight enough to appose the wound edges. In the muscle layers suture should be spaced about one every 2 cm, while in the skin slightly more are advised
- single layer closure (see Figure 3.9b) is faster but less cosmetically pleasing, and any wound infection is liable to be more severe
- avoid leaving any dead space

Discussion
The above technique achieves optimal apposition of peritoneum, musculature and skin, and the cosmetic result is pleasing. Any buried deep sutures should be of absorbable material in view of probable human consumption of the carcass.

Intra-abdominal and systemic antibiotherapy
Routine intra-abdominal medication is unnecessary. Peritonitis is controlled by systemic medication if the animal is not salvaged at once. Drainage of purulent exudate is unlikely to help control of an active process.

Intra-abdominal medication should be considered only if infection has been introduced into the peritoneal cavity. Suitable drugs include antibiotic aqueous solutions or oleaginous suspensions as carriers. Intramammary cerate preparations should not be inserted into the abdominal cavity or body wall. The most effective prophylactic medication is systemic injection of ceftiofur, penicillin, oxytetracycline hydrochloride or a single injection of long-acting oxytetracycline (see Section 1.12, p. 44).

Complications of exploratory laparotomy

- intra-operative collapse: occasionally a weak subject undergoing a 'last-ditch' exploratory laparotomy collapses during intra-abdominal exploration causing gross peritoneal contamination. Such cattle, usually thin cows, are unsuitable subjects for surgery, and should be excluded on pre-operative clinical examination (see Section 1.4, pp. 10–11)
- wound dehiscence: results from non-sterile, excessively fine material, material traumatised by forceps before or during insertion, massive wound swelling causing tearing out of sutures, and development of a subcutaneous or subperitoneal abscess, or emphysema

  Treatment of wound dehiscence: in such cases any remaining (non-functional) suture material should be removed and the wound cleansed, débrided and resutured if no infection is present, leaving a 3–10 cm opening in the ventral commissure for drainage purposes.

Cases with copious purulent discharge involving a still relatively intact wound should be opened slightly, both dorsally and ventrally, to permit vigorous irrigation with dilute chlorhexidine gluconate solution (10 ml of 5% solution made up to 1 litre with clean tap water). The incision is then left to heal by secondary intention.

In the presence of considerable necrotic tissue, preliminary irrigation with dilute H_2O_2 (3%) may be useful. (N.B. this solution may spread infection between tissue layers.) See Section 1.13.

3.4 Rumenotomy

Indications

- removal of foreign body in traumatic reticulitis or reticuloperitonitis
- gross severe rumen overload ('grain overload') involving acidosis following sudden ingestion of large volume of concentrates (barley etc.), and rarely, recent ingestion of toxic plant material (e.g. yew). Latter is usually fatal
- exploratory surgery, e.g. in chronic intermittent rumen tympany

Traumatic reticulitis

Incidence

Traumatic reticulitis is usually encountered sporadically in cattle over two years old, though occasionally farmers may experience a series of cases in a few weeks or months, associated with ingestion of particular batch of feed. Cases are more common in indoor winter feeding period on hay or silage.

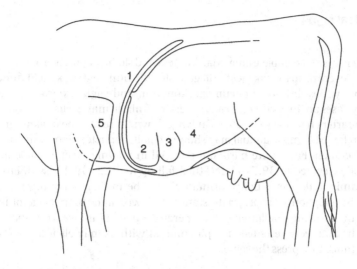

Figure 3.10 Sagittal section at diaphragmatic area, seen from left.
1. diaphragm; 2. reticulum; 3. cranial part of ventral sac of rumen; 4. rumen;
5. heart.

Aetiology

Most foreign bodies ingested by cattle fail to penetrate rumino-reticular wall
and remain in rumen (small stones etc.) or are eventually voided in faeces.
Long metallic foreign bodies such as pieces of wire, needles or nails (typically
chopped wire strands from decomposing lorry or car tyres, or rusting fencing)
and rarely broom bristles etc., are thrown forwards by ruminal-reticular contractions into the honeycombed reticulum which contracts and the foreign
body may penetrate the mucosa. Common site is the cranial and ventral
reticular wall. Penetration to depth of 5–7 mm results in perforation of the
visceral peritoneum, and point then traumatises opposing parietal peritoneum,
usually the diaphragm and occasionally the abdominal wall, spleen or liver
(see Figure 3.10).

Pain arises from irritation to peritoneum and may be temporary, the
foreign body dropping back loose into the reticular wall or lumen, either
to repenetrate at another point or to pass further down the alimentary
tract where further trouble is most unlikely. At site of penetration an acute
localised inflammatory reaction with exudate becomes slowly organised
as an adhesion, or abscess. In others cases the foreign body slowly advances
further, persistent pain is apparent for several days, and the foreign body
may eventually enter the thorax and heart, liver, spleen or abdominal wall.
Sequelae of reticular foreign body penetration and their signs are multiple,
potentially fatal, and are discussed on page 91.

Clinical signs

Acute stage

Sudden onset of complete anorexia, dullness and slightly apprehensive appearance, severe drop in milk yield, stiff gait, slightly hunched back, mild ruminal tympany, possibly some pneumoperitoneum, and slight expiratory grunt. Many cases are in early post-partum period. Animal may prefer to stand with forequarters relatively elevated. On lying down there may be obvious grunt. When forced to move animal may show stiff gait, abducted elbows and tucked up abdomen. Faeces are hard and reduced in volume. Rectal temperature initially elevated to 39.7–41.1°C then falling to 39.2–39.4°C with little or no ruminoreticular activity. Urination may be initially suspended due to pain in adoption of appropriate stance, followed later by passage of large volume of urine. Ballottement or percussion of cranioventral abdomen may be markedly resented, and pinching of withers may elicit a grunt and reluctance to depress the spine.

Chronic stage

This starts five to seven days after acute stage and is not striking or characteristic. Appetite is improved but not normal, often preferring concentrates to roughage. Slight ruminal tympany is evident. Stance is almost normal although slight stiffness is possible, while ruminal movements are present but of reduced intensity.

Diagnosis

Usually easy in early stages of acute case and is based on sudden onset of pyrexia, localised pain and ruminal stasis. In chronic cases diagnosis is often difficult. Sporadic episodic flare-ups occur with persistent moderate pyrexia, abdominal pain, anorexia and lowered milk yield. Such recurrent attacks justify exploratory laparotomy and rumenotomy. Sixty per cent of reticular punctures completely recover spontaneously, 30% remain as localised areas of chronic peritonitis, and 10% develop serious sequelae.

Radiography, ultrasonography, laparoscopy, peritoneoscopy, abdominocentesis, haematology (leucocytosis with left shift) and metal detector are ancillary aids to diagnose traumatic reticulitis. Such specialised diagnostic methods have obvious limitations even in the difficult chronic case:

- ultrasonography permits visualisation of fibrin and exudate in the abdominal cavity and reduction of the rate and intensity of ruminal contractions
- laparoscopy – expensive, time-consuming and difficult as it requires the cow to be in dorsal recumbency
- radiography – powerful equipment required and interpretation may be difficult
- abdominocentesis nonspecific as any elevated protein and WBC count may be due to other causes of peritonitis

- metal detector – non-specific for penetration, only positive with ferrous material, and false positives with cobalt and magnesium, bullets, slow release anthelmintics
- haematology – raised white cell count possibly due to other causes

Conservative treatment

Often, as signs are assessed over a few days, conservative medical treatment is instituted; forequarters should be elevated 45 cm with boarding or earth, and systemic antibiotic therapy given for three days. Magnetic probangs (Eisenhut model) and magnets have given disappointing therapeutic results. Many cases respond completely, some temporarily, to any conservative treatment.

Signs resulting from sequelae of traumatic reticuloperitonitis

- intrathoracic penetration: quite common, usually causing traumatic pericarditis (see Figure 3.10). Obvious illness about one week or more after episode of vague indigestion. Signs of congestive cardiac failure (CCF) include ventral oedema, fast pulse, distended jugular veins and localised pain. Such cases usually die within one to two weeks. Less commonly, intrathoracic foreign body causes localised abscessation in one lung lobe with chronic suppurative pneumonia and localised thoracic pain. Occasional entry into pleural space leads to fibrinopurulent pleuritis. Rarely reaction occurs in the mediastinum, and if extensive can cause pressure on heart sufficient to cause CCF (i.e. pericarditis may not be the cause of CCF)
- intra-abdominal penetration: results in hepatic, reticular, omasal or abomasal wall adhesions and a more or less localised peritonitis. Signs are vague with dullness, pyrexia and anterior abdominal pain. Splenic abscession may cause septicaemia and pyaemic spread to other organs. In rare cases abscess develops over lower body wall and penetrates skin, discharging foreign body as well as pus
- chronic reticular adhesions and abscesses: may be very extensive and involve vagal nerve supply to rumen. Usually animal returns to near-normal health, but some cases develop syndrome of chronic ruminal distension or Hoflund syndrome (see Section 3.15, pp. 129–130).

Technique of rumenotomy

Rumenotomy is the preferred treatment for acute traumatic reticuloperitonitis, and is also indicated in suspicious cases of chronic disease which are non-responsive to conservative treatment including chemotherapy, administration of a permanent magnet, and management change.

Site is in left flank as described in exploratory laparotomy (see Section 3.2, pp. 79–84). Length of incision should be 18–25 cm, but varies somewhat with the particular technique selected to control possible contamination by ruminal contents:

- Weingart frame – incision as above
- McLintock cuff – incision length 16 cm
- suture of ruminal wall to parietal peritoneum – no critical length. Ensure in all cases that dorsal commissure of incision is about 8 cm ventral to lateral extremity of lumbar transverse processes.

Having entered abdominal cavity (see Section 3.2, pp. 79–84 for technique) and before making rumenotomy incision check several points:

- appearance of visible parietal and visceral (ruminal) peritoneum, e.g. roughening indicative of acute or chronic peritonitis
- explore right side of abdominal cavity first
- presence of excessive abdominal fluid: pass hand ventrally, and excessive abdominal fluid is easily obtained in handfuls, i.e. repeated volumes of 20–50 ml. A greyish-yellow colour with floccules of pus is evidence of acute or chronic peritonitis
- presence of adhesions between reticulum, and diaphragm and adjacent viscera: indicative of past or present foreign body penetration. For assessment of age of adhesions see p. 84.

To avoid potential contamination of the abdominal cavity by ruminal contents, the ruminal lumen is either exteriorised (Weingart frame or McLintock cuff) or the abdominal cavity is sealed off from the rumen by temporary insertion of a continuous suture. The preferred method is the Weingart frame.

Weingart frame method (Figure 3.11)

The stainless steel frame (size 27 × 18 cm) is used with two vulsellum forceps (23 cm) fixed with single hooks near the junction of blade and handle, and with six small (7 cm) tenaculum hooks. Having entered abdominal cavity:

- screw the Weingart frame into the dorsal commissure of the skin incision
- push ruminal contents inwards at intended rumenotomy incision
- grasp rumen wall dorsally and about 15 cm ventrally with the two pairs of forceps, exteriorise and fix to two rings at top and bottom of frame. This brings out the rumen but does not yet prevent contamination
- place a sterile cloth or rubber drape or shroud completely around the exteriorised rumen between the frame and the abdominal wall
- incise the rumen just below the dorsal forceps
- insert one of the small ruminal hooks into the ruminal mucosa near the edge, pull back and clip the rumen onto edge of the frame at eleven o'clock position, followed by another at one o'clock

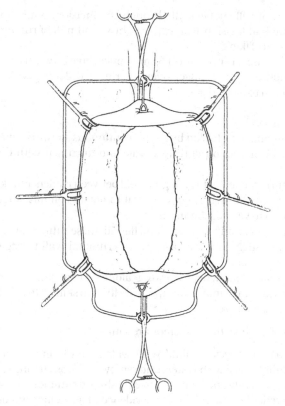

Figure 3.11 Weingart frame placed to exteriorise and fix ruminal wall with six hooks and two vulsellum forceps.

- extend ruminal incision ventrally to an appropriate length for entry of the arm and attach rumen to frame with four further hooks at nine, three, then seven and five o'clock positions. The ruminal lumen is now effectively isolated from the abdominal cavity

McLintock cuff method
This method is equally efficient but presents greater problems with sterilisation of equipment, and rubber components eventually perish.

- a special rubber cloth with everted stiff cuff surrounding the abdominal incision is placed over the flank
- exteriorise rumen and make 2.5 cm incision in upper position
- insert rubber-covered hook which is held temporarily by a non-sterile assistant
- extend incision ventrally to 10–11 cm length

- insert rim of stiff rubber cuff through the incision, whereupon the lips of the ruminal incision will grip it tightly, and pull of rumen draws rim against skin of flank
- place a thin rubber sheet with 15 cm elliptical hole between rumen and skin
- place another, similar sheet over the rim and double back the edge of ruminal cuff to form a seal

Suture method

- suture ruminal wall to skin by simple continuous suture of non-absorbable material (4 metric) on cutting needle and to rumen with Cushing-type pattern
- after suturing, check site for a good seal between rumen and skin
- incise rumen starting 2.5 cm ventral to dorsal commissure and ending 3 cm dorsal to ventral commissure
- if rumen is not relatively empty and flaccid, these sutures can possibly tear out, and in such doubtful cases suture ruminal wall to edge of parietal peritoneal incision
- for easy handling when working alone, dorsal and ventral parts of exteriorised rumen may be temporarily fixed to skin by towel clips (13 cm) for suturing purposes

Regardless of method, the next steps are similar:

- siphon off any excessive fluid with wide bore (3 cm internal diameter) plastic tubing filled with water, and remove any obstructing solid material
- pass arm cranially and ventrally over U-shaped ruminoreticular pillar and explore reticulum methodically. Evidence of adhesions already palpated during intra-abdominal exploration may lead hand to a particular area otherwise make initial rapid examination of the reticular floor, then of cranial wall
- identify and examine the cardia, oesophageal groove, and the reticulo-omasal opening as well as the medial wall: touching of reticulo-omasal orifice should provoke contraction
- remove loose reticular foreign bodies, but search specifically for pointed longitudinal foreign body lodged in secondary reticular cells between the secondary crests which characterise this organ
- search with fingertips as only 1 cm or less length of foreign body may protrude into lumen. In other cases it can subsequently be confirmed that the foreign body has passed right through the reticular wall
- it may be helpful to elevate the reticular wall with fingers to assess the presence of adhesions out of reach on parietal surface, e.g. right side
- palpate reticular wall also for discrete abscesses
- if penetrating foreign body is found, and before its removal note depth and direction of penetration to consider the likely structures damaged at this time. This aids prognosis. The wisdom of puncturing and draining

reticular or ruminal wall abscesses from the ruminoreticular lumen should be carefully assessed
- use a magnet to retrieve loose ferrous material more easily
- consider placing permanent magnet into reticulum

Difficulty in reaching furthest points for exploration due to physical size of the animal or surgeon may be partially overcome by elevation of the forequarters, causing reticulum to drop back slightly, or indirect pressure on reticular area by upward pressure on the xiphoid region by an assistant (or two, using a wooden plank).

Ruminal medication may be given after exploration of the reticulum. Although awkward to obtain (unless from slaughterhouse) fresh ruminal contents quickly normalise the flora.

Treatment of adhesions
- chronic adhesions: there is usually little or no benefit from breaking down chronic adhesions, which tend to reform very rapidly
- recent adhesions: do not break down since they may mask and surround an abscess cavity

Closure of ruminal incision
Method varies slightly with the method of fixation, but in all instances two layers of inversion sutures should be placed. These should be:

- continuous Cushing inversion suture of 4 metric PDS
- continuous Lembert inversion suture of similar material

Weingart frame method
- remove the small ruminal clips and clean the peritoneal surface before and after placing the two suture layers, and clean again before releasing large forceps, permitting rumen to drop back into abdominal cavity

McLintock cuff method
- remove the two rubber sheets, avoiding contamination, pull out rumen and internal cuff further from body wall and apply foam-rubber edged special rumen clamp under rim of tube which is then removed
- clamp then rests on flank with ruminal edges safely fixed and the contaminated surfaces may be easily cleaned, and the two layer suture (Cushing or Lembert type) placed in position

Suture method
- after initial cleansing of exposed ruminal surface insert two layers of sutures and then carry out thorough cleansing of the surfaces
- débride any contaminated tissue from the body wall musculature
- remove the circumferential peritoneal suture

Intra-abdominal medication is not specifically indicated. Closure of abdominal wall has been previously described (see Section 3.3, pp. 85–88). All cases should receive systemic antibiotic therapy for three to ten days.

Prevention of traumatic reticulitis

Prevention may be difficult to achieve. However, advent of plastic bale twine and disappearance of wire has removed a major source of potential foreign bodies. Encourage at-risk farms to remove ferrous and other potentially hazardous materials from field and lane edges (e.g. during hedge-trimming).

Consider, where economically justified (especially AI centres and pedigree stock farms), use of permanent magnets (Bovivet® ruminal magnet, Kruuse) given orally, from one year old onwards. Best type is cage model in which a plastic case surrounds magnet so that most ferrous material lies within the grooves, avoiding any contact with the reticular epithelium (Hannover model cage magnet super 11). Magnet appears an effective prophylactic measure.

3.5 Temporary rumen fistulation

Indications

Chronic recurrent ruminal tympany usually occurs in calves of three to nine months. Condition causes unthriftiness resulting from reduced feed intake. Fistula affords symptomatic relief and is rapidly produced. Alternatively, self-retaining disposable calf trocar (Buff spiral model, 11 cm Kruuse) may be used for a few days, but requires to be cleaned regularly with metallic trocar to avoid blockage.

Aetiology of recurrent tympany in calves

Often caused by inadequate fibre intake and poor rumen development. Occasionally there is obstruction of thoracic oesophagus and/or cardia by external pressure by mediastinal lymphadenopathy, which may be sequel to chronic pneumonic pathology. Stomach tube can often be passed without any difficulty, so excluding possibility of mechanical stricture or stenosis.

Signs

Slight but progressive loss of condition associated with more or less permanent overdistension of rumen. Many such calves eventually recover spontaneously. Rumination is usually unaffected.

Technique

- paravertebral analgesia (T13, L1, see Section 1.8, pp. 22–24) or local infiltration analgesia (see Section 1.7, pp. 26–27). Site is upper left paralumbar fossa, one third of distance from last rib to external angle of ilium
- clip skin over site 10 × 7 cm and disinfect
- pass stomach tube to relieve any tympany

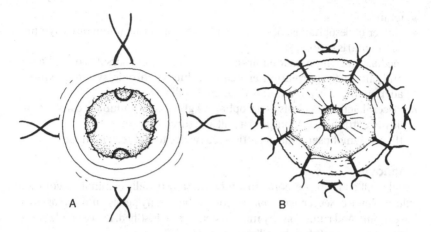

Figure 3.12 One technique of suturing rumen to body wall to create ruminal fistula. A. four mattress sutures from ruminal wall to skin; B. eight simple sutures to overlap rumen over skin edges; Fistula of appropriate size may then be made.

- remove oval section of skin 4 × 2 cm, and split muscularis by blunt dissection (scissors)
- pick up peritoneum with Allis forceps, incise, and grasp
- exteriorise underlying ruminal wall with second Allis forceps
- place sutures (polyamide) between skin and rumen using interrupted horizontal mattress pattern or simple continuous stuture for initial fixation (see Figure 3.12a)

   Alternatively, a screw trocar (Buff model) may be inserted through flank for several weeks as needed. Problems can occur: lumen blockage, displacement out of rumen, peritonitis
- incise rumen (3 cm) and place four or eight simple sutures to overlap rumen and skin margin (see Figure 3.12)
- if thought necessary, convert slit into oval by removing portion of wall slightly smaller than the previously resected skin

This ruminal incision usually heals in three to five weeks following fibrous tissue proliferation and stricture. A permanent fistula requires a ruminal incision at least 6 cm long.

Chronic ruminal tympany in adult cattle

Aetiology
Causes include:
- chronic reticulitis commonly with adhesion formation, with signs reflecting poor ruminal contractility subsequent to vagal nerve injury (see Figure 3.22)

- tetanus
- cancer of oesophagus, oesophageal groove or cardia (alimentary lymphosarcoma) is rare cause
- mediastinal lymph node enlargement, nodes resting dorsal to oesophagus and effectively preventing erutcation, due to chronic systemic lymphadenopathy, e.g. pneumonia, or actinobacillosis
- visceral actinobacillosis of oesophageal groove, reticulum or cardia, usually in cattle between one and a half and three years old
- thymic lymphosarcoma in cattle aged twelve to eighteen months

Diagnosis
Usually difficult. Non-response to antibiotherapy usually eliminates actinobacillosis. Some cases recover spontaneously, but many persist and exploratory laparotomy and rumenotomy may sometimes be justified, i.e. valuable cattle with considerable future breeding potential.

Treatment and prognosis
Apart from actinobacillosis (iodides and/or antibiotics, e.g. streptomycin) treatment of chronic ruminal tympany in adult cattle is usually unsuccessful. Creation of semi-permanent ruminal fistula generally fails to alleviate primary condition. Prognosis is poor.

3.6 Left displacement of abomasum

Anatomy
The abomasum normally lies on the abdominal floor, and its relations depend on the degree of distension of rumen, reticulum and omasum, and their contraction. The abomasum has the fundic and pyloric regions. The distinction between fundus and corpus (body) is imprecise and of no clinical interest. The narrower pyloric part passes transversely and possibly slightly craniad along the right body wall, to pass into the pylorus which lies caudal and lateral to the ventral part of the omasum beneath ribs 11–12.

Aetiology
Left displacement of abomasum (LDA), right dilatation and displacement (RDA), and abomasal volvulus probably have a common aetiology despite differing symptomatology. LDA aetiology involves abomasal fundus hypomotility and hypotonicity resulting in delayed emptying. Factors include:

- over-conditioning (fat) at parturition
- diet – high concentrate intake, often with high fat and/or protein, and relatively low percentage of fibre in diet
- overeating or sudden change of feed, (e.g. absence of roughage at night), other stress factors (e.g. dystocia)
- inherited factors in some strains

- rearrangement of viscera associated with parturition
- concurrent diseases (e.g. fatty liver and ketosis, metritis, mastitis, hypocalcaemia) are often associated with abomasal displacement

Signs

- dairy cattle, winter-housed period and usually within six weeks of parturition, increasing incidence today in calved heifers and calves
- relatively sudden drop in yield and selective anorexia, refusing most concentrates
- reduced or absent ruminal movements and reduced rumination
- animal fairly bright and without abdominal pain except in rare case (with peptic ulceration, perforation and acute localised peritonitis)
- mild constipation initially
- afebrile (except with secondary peritonitis or concurrent disease)
- frequently secondary ketonuria with positive Rothera's test (milk) and sweet smell in expired air
- mild hypochloraemia, hypokalaemia and slight metabolic alkalosis possible
- possible recent history of dystocia, milk fever, metritis or mastitis
- progressive and accelerating loss of condition

Diagnosis

Auscultation of left flank pathognomonic: high-pitched metallic tinkling sounds from left flank over middle area bounded by ribs 10–13. Corresponding area of resonance detected by applying stethoscope and by flicking forefinger against rib cage; echo-like sound 'steelband effect' or 'ping' is quite different from dullness appreciated with rumen closely applied to left body wall. In doubtful case ballotte ventral ruminal sac with right knee while auscultating left flank over ribs 10–12 (greater frequency of abnormal sounds).

Occasionally a slight distention of dorsocranial part of left paralumbar fossa just behind rib 13 results from severe abomasal tympany.

Rarely can LDA be detected on rectal examination as a tympanitic viscus between left dorsal sac of rumen and left flank.

Differential diagnosis

Differential diagnosis of left flank resonance: hypotonic form of vagus indigestion may reveal peritoneal fluid and gas

In rare difficult cases a 'liptac test' can be used to confirm the diagnosis. An 8 cm 14 gauge needle is pushed through the body wall into the centre of the area defined by a 'ping'. Centesis is used to collect some fluid. A pH less than 3.5 indicates a displaced abomasum; a pH greater than 5.5 suggests the 'ping' comes from the rumen. An orogastric tube can also be passed into the rumen to help differentiate a rumen 'ping' from that due to LDA. By ultrasonography the LDA can be visualised as a fluid- and gas-filled viscus covering the rumen.

Conservative technique

Indicated in recent cases where economic factors (cost of surgery) are important. Treatment is primarily replacement by rolling.

- cast cow on right side (Reuff's method, one person restraining head, two on ropes)
- turn over on to left side and while turning ballotte ventral abdominal wall firmly in an attempt to move abomasum into midline position, using knee to push anti-clockwise
- alternatively cast cow on back in dorsal recumbency and move from 45° right lateral to 45° left lateral position, 'shaking' abomasum back into normal position
- finally, in either rolling method, turn cow into left lateral recumbency and maintain in this position for five to ten minutes to permit organ to evacuate excessive gas
- check absence of abomasum from left side on auscultation and finger percussion
- inject calcium and dextrose i.v.
- re-introduce concentrates slowly over one week period to cows corrected of LDA by rolling
- encourage maximal exercise in this period

Some cases of LDA corrected by rolling may at once or soon become cases of RDA. Many others have a recurrence of LDA within 48 hours and require rolling again or surgery. Success rate of rolling is about 20%.

Surgical technique (LDA)

Numerous methods of surgical correction have been described since the first reports of LDA, around 1948, in Scotland.

Some options of sites and fixation techniques include:

- standing or recumbent surgery
- left or right, or bilateral flank incision
- paracostal, paramedian or midline incision
- fixation of abomasum to right flank or ventral body wall by intra-abdominal approach
- left flank laparoscopic approach and right paramedian fixation (not discussed further)
- percutaneous fixation from abdominal cavity (Utrecht technique)
- midline percutaneous fixation through 'blind' suture, or (popular) toggle technique

Advantages and disadvantages of various surgical sites are listed in Table 3.1. Personal preference varies enormously.

Table 3.1 Surgical correction of left displaced abomasum: different methods.

Incision site	Right flank	Left flank (Utrecht)	Right and left flank	Midline/paramedian	Paracostal	Percutaneous fixation (toggle)
Anaesthesia	paravertebral or local infiltration	paravertebral or local infiltration	paravertebral or local infiltration	sedation (xylazine + local infiltration)	sedation (xylazine + local infiltration)	sedation (xylazine)
Ease of decompression	+	++	++	(+)	(+)	N/A
Ease of reposition	++	+	++	(+)	(+)	(+)
Area of abomasal fixation	pylorus	fundus	fundus or pylorus	fundus	fundus	fundus
Remarks	relatively unphysiological position of fixation, minimal stress	technical problems in inexperienced hands; rumenotomy also possible	2 surgeons; added time and expense; rumenotomy also possible	possible restraint problems; good wound closure essential	haemorrhage and wound healing problems	good, assistant needed, fast cheap, but risk of misdirected fixation (e.g. rumen)
Personal preferences of authors						
(ADW)	1	2	3	5	6	4
(GSJ)	1	3	5	2	6	4
(AS)	1	2[a] 3[b]	0	3[b]	0	4[c]

Abbreviations (+) = usually spontaneous decompression and reposition following recumbency
[a] = antepartum LDA; [b] = long standing LDA, [c] = low value cow

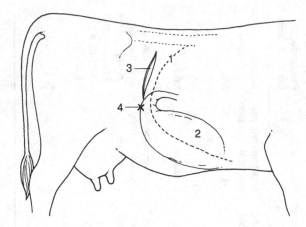

Figure 3.13 Diagram of right flank of cow to show site of laparotomy incision for right flank abomasopexy.
1. rib 13; 2. abomasal fundus and body; 3. flank incision; 4. abomasopexy site (x) sutured to body wall.

Right flank approach
- paravertebral analgesia T13, L1 and L2
- skin preparation for aseptic surgery and drape
- paracostal skin incision 15–20 cm long starting 10 cm below tip of L2 transverse process and 4 cm behind last rib (see Figure 3.13)
- entry into abdomen as previously described (see Section 3.2) with blunt separation of muscle layers and incision of transverse fascia and peritoneum, extended to permit comfortable entry of one hand (13 cm)
- make thorough manual exploration of abdominal cavity (see Figure 3.8); then insert the left hand, passing it behind the caudal edge of the greater omentum and over to the left side of the abdominal cavity, directed initially towards the lower part of the wing of the ileum, ventral to descending colon and mesocolon and the left perirenal fat mass
- appreciate the displaced abomasum interposed between a relatively small rumen and the left body wall (abomasum may extend two-thirds or often further up the left flank)
- check the palpable area of the abomasum for any roughness (peritonitis) and adhesions to the left flank. Peritonitis is probably due to a perforated peptic ulcer. It may prove difficult to reposition the abomasum, either by pushing it down or pulling on the greater omentum from the right side, before evacuating most abomasal gas

- decompress the abomasum by inserting wide bore needle (2.1 metric, approximately 2 mm internal diameter), 45° to abomasal wall firmly attached to plastic tubing, into the dorsocaudal part of the abomasum with the free end of the tubing (length approximately 2 m) held outside the animal and evacuate air
- maintain needle firmly in place while gently pushing the viscus ventrally with palm of hand
- anticipate that gas will be evacuated over five minutes (volume 5–15 litres) until the abomasal wall is relatively flaccid and almost out of reach, low down on the left side
- remove needle and tubing, carefully avoiding contamination of abdominal cavity by abomasal fluid in tubing
- place left hand onto dorsal aspect of abomasum and push it down towards midline
- pass left hand along right body wall with palm against rib cage to midline, midway between xiphisternum and umbilicus
- turn hand through 180° in clockwise direction, and grasp the greater omentum and abomasum now lying in midline
- hold this mass firmly and pull upwards, if necessary in a series of gentle jerking movements, and identify abomasum through right flank wound
- identify the abomasal pyloric region visually: pale pink-grey and well delineated from adjacent insertion of greater omentum, it is firm and cannot be easily traumatised by the fingers
- if not visible through flank incision repeat midline grasping process; abomasum is easily drawn into right flank using this technique
- release abomasum and greater omentum temporarily for confirmatory manual check of left side for absence of abomasum
- check remainder of cranial abdominal cavity (liver, reticulum, diaphragm) by rapid manual exploration
- suture greater omentum to parietal peritoneum and transversalis muscle in closure of flank
- pull suture tight and tie off, ensuring that no small intestine inadvertently becomes trapped. Place second suture about 3 cm dorsal to the first
- alternatively suture lateral pyloric wall of abomasum and several centimetres of adjacent omentum to body wall. Needle should be about 4.5 cm long, semi-curved and round-bodied, threaded with 5 metric monofilament nylon
- close abdominal incision in routine manner (see Section 3.3, pp. 86–87)
- give systemic antibiotic therapy for one to three days.

Improvement is usually seen after two to three days with an increased appetite for concentrate. Prognosis in uncomplicated cases is excellent (95%).

Complications

Post-operative complications include:

- peritonitis due to non-sterile technique or leakage of abomasal fluid causing peritonitis or abscessation in the flank wound
- recurrence resulting from breakage of the abomasal flank pexy site suture before development of adhesion formation
- wound dehiscence, usually ventrally
- functional stenosis possible after tacking pyloric part of abomasum instead of greater omentum

Left flank approach

Thought not widely practised in the UK and North America, this (Utrecht) technique deserves greater recognition for its simplicity.

- make left paracostal incision as for exploratory laparotomy (incision 3, Fig. 3.6)
- explore abdominal cavity and identity LDA
- evacuate gas from abomasum with needle as previously described, or by simple pressure (some surgeons prefer to place suture first, then evacuate gas)
- thread 1.5 m length of non-absorbable suture material (polyamide polymer 4 gauge) onto straight triangular 8 cm needle, and insert needle through greater omentum and wall, but not lumen of abomasal body in series of five to six continuous sutures, each 3 cm apart (Ford interlocking) (see Figure 3.14)
- push semi-flaccid abomasum down towards midline
- insert needle through body wall slightly right of the abdominal midline, midway between xiphisternum and umbilicus (site indicated by assistant's finger pressure on skin)
- ensure needle is pulled through skin to exterior by assistant, and that end of suture material is retained in artery forceps dangling beneath the abdominal wall
- with second needle threaded from distal end of same suture material push needle through ventral body wall 3–10 cm caudal to first point; assistant can again indicate correct site
- assistant then ties suture on skin of ventral abdominal wall, (placing roll of bandage below suture) while surgeon ensures that abomasum is held firmly against ventral parietal peritoneum so preventing interposition of greater omentum or jejunal loops
- close abdominal flank in routine manner and give systemic antibiotics for one to three days
- remove abomaso-omental skin sutures with scissors after two weeks, when firm adhesion of greater omentum and abomasum to body wall has formed

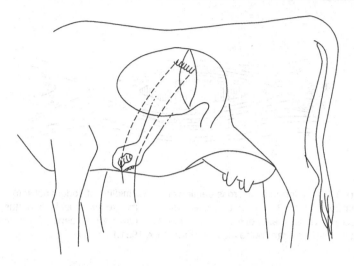

Figure 3.14 Abomasopexy from the left side using Utrecht method. Continuous suture has been placed through greater omentum at insertion onto abomasum in left flank. Suture is then pushed through ventral body wall just right of midline using a long straight needle.

Midline approach

Reposition and fixation present few difficulties. Surgery may be performed under sedation (xylazine, i.v. or i.m.) and local analgesia, or under GA. Animal should be supported by straw bales laterally, and hind legs should be roped away from operative site. A stockman, restraining head, keeps forelegs away from surgical field, operator's head and hands.

- incision is midway between umbilicus and xiphisternum approximately 15 cm long if visual exploration is required, or 11 cm if manipulation and deep sutures are to be inserted by palpation alone
- incise skin, subcutaneous fat and linea alba (approximately 7 mm thick) with scalpel (see Figure 3.15)
- note small amount of subperitoneal fat overlying peritoneum, which is incised with scalpel and lengthened with straight scissors
- explore abdomen thoroughly with sweeping movement
- pass hand to left side to identify displaced abomasum or (if reposition has already occurred, which is likely) ventral sac of rumen
- follow greater omentum from insertion onto left longitudinal groove of rumen over towards midline to identify body of abomasum
- briefly exteriorise abomasal body for identification

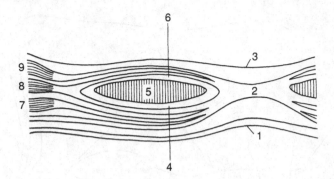

Figure 3.15   Diagrammatic cross-section of ventral midline of abdominal wall.
1. skin; 2 *linea alba*; 3. peritoneum; 4. external sheath of rectus muscle; 5. rectus
muscle; 6. internal sheath of rectus muscle; 7. external oblique muscle; 8. internal
oblique muscle; 9. transverse muscle. (From Cox, 1981.)

- suture abomasum to peritoneum and vental abdominal musculature
  enclosing with each suture about 2 cm width of abomasal body (using
  polyamide polymer 4 metric or PDS)
- ensure that sutures do not penetrate lumen (danger of fistula or tearing
  out with risk of fatal peritonitis) but include serosa and muscularis
- continuous peritoneal suture, carefully tightening whole length before
  tying off
- suture *linea alba* (most important supporting layer of abdominal wall) with
  simple interrupted sutures of PGA 5 or 6 metric on semi-curved cutting
  edge needle 5 cm long
- bury this layer with continuous layer of subcutaneous sutures of PGA
  4 metric
- suture skin in horizontal everted mattress pattern with monofilament nylon
- systemic antibiotics for one to three days
- remove skin sutures after ten days.

Percutaneous fixation (toggle or bar suture)
A rapid and simple technique of abomasal fixation avoiding the need for
expensive laparotomy which has found widespread acceptance over the last
twenty years. Following diagnosis of an uncomplicated LDA the steps are:

- clip and disinfect the ventral abdomen to right of midline between xiphoid
  and umbilicus, marking position of right abdominal vein
- give 45–50 mg xylazine i.v. and cast cow (e.g. by Reuff's method) on right
  side
- turn quickly into dorsal recumbency and extend and tie hind legs, place
  straw bales against flanks for stability

- assistant kneels in front of udder from left side while surgeon confirms by auscultation the presence of tympanitic abomasum ventrally
- trocar and cannula (Kruuse UK Ltd, Jorgensen Labs, Colorado, USA) are inserted firmly through skin, musculature and peritoneum about a hand's-width caudal to xiphoid and similar distance right of midline (see Figure 3.16)
- pull out trocar and insert toggle, having confirmed entry into abomasum (gas always escapes and acidic pH can be checked with dipstick)

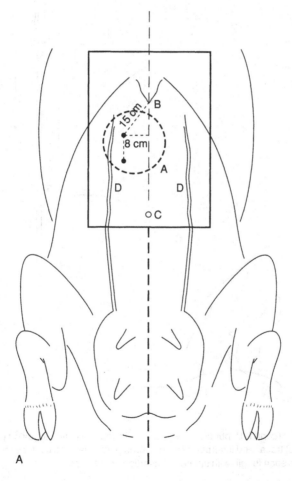

Figure 3.16 Abomasal 'toggling' procedure through skin of ventral cranial body wall. A. ventral view showing puncture sites distal to xiphisternum (B), and to right side between midline and right mammary vein (D).

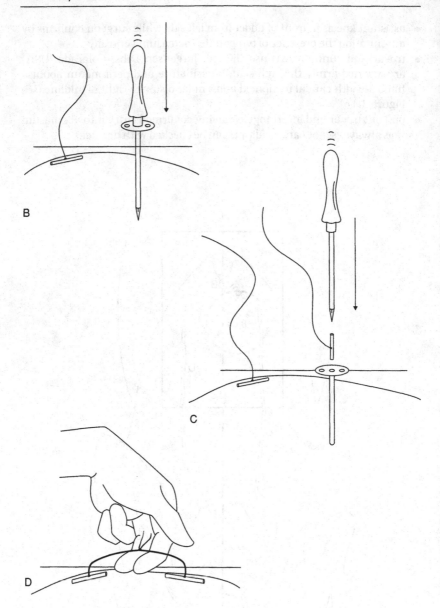

Figure 3.16   (*cont'd*) B. puncture by trocar and canula with first toggle in place;
C. removal of trocar and insertion of toggle through canula; D. tying together of
sutures from each toggle with space for insertion of two fingers.

- assistant holds toggle suture with forceps
- remove cannula and rapidly repeat trocarisation and toggle insertion two fingers'-width caudal or cranial to first site
- permit most gas to escape
- tie two sutures together allowing several centimetres of play (see Figure 3.16d)
- turn cow onto sternum slowly and allow to stand
- prophylactic systemic antibiotic cover
- post-operative visit about two to five days later to check abomasal position and any concurrent disease problems.

This percutaneous procedure requires two assistants and must be performed quickly as the abomasum can rapidly deflate once the cow is on her back. If unsuccessful, a standing surgery can be done. The major hazards, apart from personal injury from poor restraint, are the risk of puncturing rumen, fixation of abomasum too close to the pylorus and tearing of the abomasal wall by the suture, all potentially resulting in peritonitis.

The easiest cases tend to be cows with obvious 'pings' in the left flank at first clinical examination, since abomasum remains gas-filled relatively longer. The technique clearly does not permit examination of other abdominal viscera for concurrent disease (e.g. chronic adhesions, hepatic abscessation).

Discussion of surgical techniques

Some surgical problems and their proposed solutions are:

- inability to locate abomasum – if encountered during right flank approach it may be necessary to perform left flank incision, especially in case of inexperienced surgeon
- inability to break down left flank adhesions of abomasum to body wall – adhesions may be out of reach in right flank approach, again necessitating left flank laparotomy, or they may be too firm to break down due to their longstanding and extensive nature. Beware of breaking down recent adhesions which may result in exposure of abomasal lumen through a perforated ulcer. Such complications are rare (< 5%)
- inability to replace abomasum from right flank approach – as long as midline structures are firmly grasped in palm of hand, avoiding risk of puncturing abomasum or of tearing omentum with finger tips, repeated gentle traction is harmless. Check that hand is grasping structures about 20 cm caudal to xiphisternum
- inability to identify pyloric region – identify caudal portion of abomasal wall adjacent to greater omentum, then pass hand dorsally, and eventually area can be identified where abomasum is about 3 cm wide and where

small lobes of greater and lesser omental fat overlap the abomasal border. Abomasum is thicker and denser at this point (pyloric antrum), which is the pylorus, located below rib 10, about half-way down body wall

3.7 Right dilatation, displacement and volvulus of abomasum

Right dilatation and displacement of abomasum probably have common aetiology with LDA. Incidence is lower and RDA is not so closely related to early post-partum period. RDA can result from rolling of LDA cases, in which dilated organ is displaced a variable distance into the right flank. In some cases a cow may apparently have alternately LDA and RDA, the organ 'swinging' from one flank to the other over a period of several days. Right dilatation occasionally occurs in younger cattle and in steers.

Signs and diagnosis of RDA
- selective anorexia and gradual weight loss
- distension of low and mid right flank where auscultation reveals high pitched splashing and sometimes ringing sounds
- RDA case usually has relatively more fluid than LDA animal
- ballottement of low right flank causes loud splashing sounds but rarely any pain
- cows may show profuse watery diarrhoea
- rectal examination may reveal a smooth distended viscus on the right side cranial to pubic brim, though only the caudal and dorsal surfaces can be reached. At any time an RDA can develop into a right-sided volvulus with or without severe compromise of the local vasculature. Few cases of RDA rapidly develop volvulus but, once it occurs, condition is acute and prognosis becomes guarded within some hours. Surgery is then an emergency.

Animals with RDA may make spontaneous recovery but many become progressively duller, and some develop bradycardia. Prognosis is guarded.

Conservative treatment of RDA
Turn animal out to grass or into yard for increased exercise and maintain access to bulky fodder as high priority. Some cases respond well to general symptomatic treatment, others to metaclopromide. Recently calved cows may be given calcium borogluconate both i.v. and s.c.. Non-responsive cases of RDA remain at risk of developing abomasal volvulus. Many cases of volvulus have a retrospectively elicitable history of chronic abomasal disease. Perform surgery in valuable animals as soon as possible, i.e. before volvulus occurs.

Signs of abomasal volvulus

- abdominal emergency: cow is in shock, collapsed, with tachycardia, mild to severe cyanosis
- weakness, possible recumbency depending on chronicity, severe abdominal distension, especially on right side, with loud splashing sounds on ballottement of right flank
- rectal examination reveals large, smooth and tense-walled viscus ventrally on right side
- (optional) abdominocentesis may reveal large volume of reddish-brown fluid
- severe hypochloraemia and hypokalaemia, increased PCV, increased total protein
- metabolic alkalosis due to abomasal sequestration of acidic gastric secretion, later possibly metabolic acidosis
- abomasum may contain up to 50 litres of fluid
- volvulus causes severe and potentially fatal impairment of venous drainage of abomasum, and the wall becomes ischaemic, dark red, then blue and black, at which stage rupture is likely

Differential diagnoses include caecal dilatation and dislocation, small intestinal obstruction following volvulus or invagination, functional abomasal obstruction.

In most cases mechanical movements initially involve dorsal displacement of the greater curvature followed by counter-clockwise 180°–360° torsion of the abomasum (see Figure 3.17). Postmortem (PM) examination often fails to reveal exactly what displacement was the primary movement. Pathology reveals severe constriction of both venous and arterial supply at the junction of omasum and abomasum, as well as between reticulum and omasum. The descending duodenum is completely occluded as a result of severe stenosis following external pressure and a degree of displacement. Direction has been described as clockwise or counter-clockwise when viewed from the right side. When viewed from the rear, it has a 'spiral corkscrew-like' counter-clockwise movement.

Surgical treatment of RDA and abomasal volvulus

- correct right abomasal dilatation by right flank surgery after giving fluids and electrolytes (see Table 1.11) e.g. i.v. infusion of 10–50 litres 0.9% NaCl with dextrose or Ringer lactate to any severely deficient cases. Early case of volvulus has metabolic alkalosis, late stage is acidotic.
- make right flank paracostal incision, starting 10 cm below lumbar transverse processes
- explore abdomen to determine form of displacement and any other complications

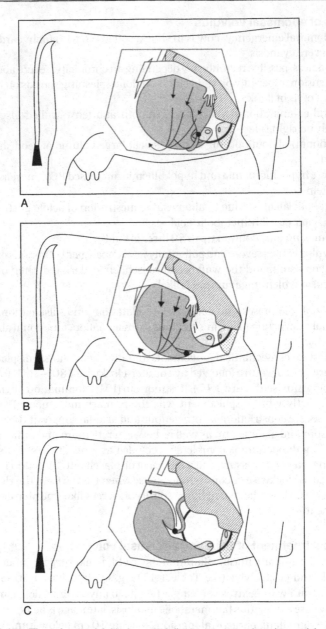

Figure 3.17   Three forms of right abomasal displacement and torsion and their manipulative correction. (From Dirksen, Gründer & Stöber, 2002.)
A. left (anti-clockwise from rear view) 360° torsion and direction of manual correction; B. left 180° torsion, and correction; C. simple right-sided abomasal displacement (possibly with up to 90° rotation). (From Dirksen, Gründer & Stöber, 2002.)

- decompress gas from abomasum. If necessary, especially in case of volvulus, fluid can be removed from the abomasum by first placing a 4–7 cm diameter circular purse string dorsally in the serosal surface of the abomasum
- make a stab incision in the centre of the purse string and insert a stomach tube quickly in the abomasum while the purse string is tied
- tighten purse-string suture which may be oversewn by one or two mattress sutures
- examine evacuated organ carefully for signs of abomasitis (diffuse hyperaemia) and ulceration (thickened areas, superficial fibrin deposition)
- locate pylorus for orientation
- correct displacement by pushing greater curvature cranially and ventrally with flat palm of hand or with forearm
- confirm that position of pyloric region and descending duodenum are normal (fundus, pyloric region, pylorus and proximal duodenum all against right abdominal wall)
- perform pyloromyotomy (optional and of controversial benefit) by longitudinal 3–4 cm incision through muscular coats of the pylorus (about 1 cm deep). If lumen is inadvertently entered, several chromic catgut sutures should be placed to bury this incision
- suture greater omentum (caudal to pylorus) to body wall (see p. 103).

Surgery of abomasal volvulus may not be indicated in cows with long-standing abomasal volvulus that are unable to rise and remain standing. Such animals should be sent to emergency slaughter on humane grounds. They often fail to pass meat inspection as the carcass may not set as the animal is usually toxic. If surgery is attempted in advanced cases, fluid therapy with i.v. lactated ringer or isotonic bicarbonate is essential before and during surgery (see Table 1.11), due to massive abomasal sequestration of Cl^-, K^+ and H^+ ions and subsequent metabolic acidosis. The prognosis is guarded or good in cases with a heart rate < 90/min, serum urea < 10 mmol/l or serum Cl^- > 85 mmol/l. Cows with abomasal volvulus of chronic nature with heart rate > 120/min and 12% dehydration have a poor prognosis for survival. The sooner abomasal volvulus is diagnosed and surgically corrected, the better the prognosis.

Surgery may be reserved for good risk standing cases and cattle where systemic antibiotic treatment has already rendered the carcass valueless for human consumption. Following the operation 20 litres of warm water containing 60 g NaCl and 30 g KCl should be given twice daily by stomach tube. It appears that abomasal torsion (up to 180°) must be distinguished from abomasal volvulus (180°–360°). The former has in the USA a guarded prognosis, when serum Cl remains above 85 mmol/l. The latter is the form usually experienced in the UK and affected cows are often recumbent at first clinical examination (see Figure 3.17).

3.8 Other abomasal conditions

Other surgical conditions of the abomasum include:

- impaction
- abomasal tympany and volvulus in calves
- ulceration (with or without perforation)

Abomasal impaction

Introduction
Impaction may be primary, as in calves following incorrect feeding with excessive roughage and an inadequate water intake. Impaction may also be secondary to surgical correction of abomasal volvulus, or to lymphosarcoma and adhesion formation in the cranial part of the abdominal cavity.

Treatment
- perform exploratory surgery through a right midflank incision
- break down abomasal contents manually
- give paraffin oil (5 litres, with 20 litres of water) by an orogastric tube once, or repeated 24 hours later

Some cases may slowly resolve. Abomasotomy through a right paramedian incision may be necessary in advanced cases.

Abomasal tympany and volvulus in calves

Signs
Seen in calves typically at six weeks to three months shortly after bucket milk feeding, signs include obvious discomfort with head extended, mild colicky signs and right flank tympany, later depression and spread of tympany to involve the left flank. Systemic signs rapidly become severe and calves can die within a few hours.

Differential diagnosis: rumen tympany (unlikely in this age group), caecal dilatation and dislocation, jejunal volvulus or intussusception

Treatment
Recumbent calves with circulatory collapse should generally be euthanised. Less severe cases:

- i.v. fluids, right paracostal or paramedian incision under local anaesthesia, in left lateral or dorsal recumbency
- exteriorise abomasum, evacuate contents by slow release of gas (tympany) or fluid
- replace organ after correction of displacement

Abomasal ulceration

Introduction

Common condition in slaughterhouse statistics, both in calves and adults. Younger cows tend to be affected within four weeks of parturition. Abomasal ulcers rarely cause significant clinical disease.

- type 1: non-perforating, minimal bleeding
- type 2: ulcer causing severe blood loss
- type 3: perforating ulcer with acute localised peritonitis
- type 4: perforating ulcer with diffuse peritonitis

Type 1 is often subclinical, while types 2 and 4 usually show clinical signs and may be fatal. In mature cows concurrent disease is often present such as mastitis, metritis and pneumonia. Abomasal ulceration tends to occur in recently calved cows (corresponding to LDA incidence) and is related to stress e.g. overcrowded yards and cubicle houses.

Signs

- abdominal pain, which is not only associated with peritonitis
- calves show abomasal dilation with ulceration (painful palpation)
- melaena and pale mucous membranes (type 2)
- pyrexia and tachycardia in cases with peritonitis
- abdominocentesis (see Section 3.16, p. 130) useful to confirm peritonitis e.g. acute fatal cases involving ruptured omental abscessation

Treatment

- type 2 ulcers require whole blood transfusion if PCV drops below 15 vols%
- treatment of peritonitis requires systemic antibiotics
- i.v. fluids
- exploration in left flank LDA: correction of left abomasal adhesions, rarely is surgical resection of ulcer necessary
- correction of primary disorder
- pyloromyotomy may improve prognosis in calves with abomasal dilation and ulceration

3.9 Caecal dilatation and dislocation

Definition and anatomy (see Figures 3.3 and 3.5)

The term dislocation refers to any twist, torsion, volvulus or retroflexion of the caecum which has a blunted round apex projecting caudally from the omental recess. Position varies with the volume of contents, floating dorsally if gas-filled or sinking with ample fluid contents. Normal caecum cannot be identified on rectal palpation.

Incidence and signs

- usually seen in adult dairy cows > 4 years old with signs rather similar to RDA for caecal dilatation and ressembling abomasal volvulus in caecal dislocation
- causes not understood and may involve hypocalcaemia and inhibitory effect of high volatile fatty acid concentrations in caecum on caecal motility
- selective anorexia (refusing concentrates) in housed or pastured cow, more frequently seen during production phase than in early lactation
- vague abdominal discomfort and pain, mild in caecal dilatation, severe in caecal dislocation
- some distension of right caudal abdominal cavity, and ballottement of upper right flank (more dorsal and caudal than in RDA and abomasal volvulus) produces sounds of fluid and gas
- faeces reduced in volume, dark, possibly covered with mucus
- rectal examination reveals little or no faeces and a mass like end of 'cob' loaf of bread 15–20 cm diameter in dilatation (see Figure 3.18a,b)
- position is relatively high on right side (dilatation), or as a distended organ (retroflexed caecal body) cranially in right ventral quadrant, or painful palpation of ileocaecal ligament (dislocation)
- dislocation of caecum produces more severe systemic signs, but disease progress is slower than in RDA and abomasal volvulus

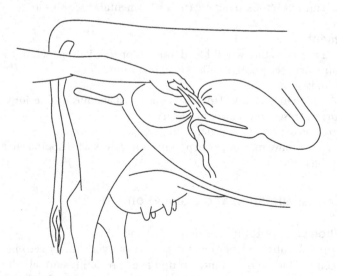

Figure 3.18(a)   Caecal torsion and retroflexion: diagrams of rectal findings. Longitudinal section through abdomen: apex of caecum and tense ileocaecal fold are palpable in caecal torsion.

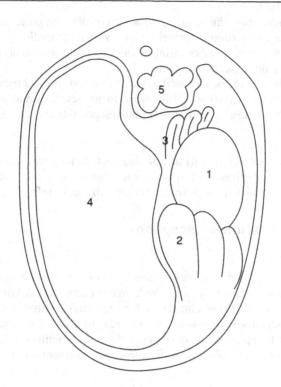

Figure 3.18(b) Transverse section through abdomen: (1) dilated body of caecum, (2) distended loops of spiral colon, and (3) sometimes also small intestine are palpable in caecal retroflexion; (4) rumen and (5) left kidney

- haematology and biochemical parameters usually normal in caecal dilatation; in caecal dislocation blood biochemistry is also normal or occasionally shows metabolic alkalosis with $\downarrow Cl^-$ and $\downarrow K^+$ caused by intestinal stasis
- differential diagnoses: RDA, abomasal volvulus, intestinal torsion around mesentery

Confirmation of diagnosis depends on right flank laparotomy.

Treatment
Medical management may be indicated in some cows with dilatation. Surgical approach:

- site of incision upper right flank, and relatively more caudal than for RDA
- exteriorise caecum and examine carefully for necrosis and commencing gangrene

- correct dislocation after drainage at apex (typhlotomy, purse-string suture placed before insertion of scalpel blade or wide-bore needle)
- massage firmer material out from intra-abdominal portion of caecum and proximal loop of ascending colon
- inspect the caecal apex for ischaemia: the easiest surgical technique is to invert such areas into caecal lumen and to oversew the area
- peri- and post-surgical systemic antibiotics, possibly i.v. or oral fluids

Prognosis
Prognosis is good (dilatation) or guarded (dislocation) and recurrence rate is up to 20%. Typhlectomy (partial caecectomy) is rarely indicated but relatively simple to perform. Cow copes well with caecum of reduced capacity.

3.10 Intestinal intussusception

Introduction
Intussusception (invagination or telescoping of bowel) occasionally affects small intestine (jejunum, ileum). Predisposing causes are unknown but the condition is not always associated with hyperperistalsis, enteritis or diarrhoea. Any age group, from calves to older cows, may be affected, but calves appear predisposed. Complete bowel obstruction results. Sometimes a double intussusception (five layers of bowel wall superimposed on each side) develops.

Signs
- sudden onset of acute abdominal pain
- groaning, kicking at belly, alternately lying and standing, paddling of hind legs
- within 12 hours acute signs are succeeded by dullness, anorexia, precipitous drop in milk yield (as in traumatic reticulitis)
- initial tachycardia (heart rate 120/min) disappears, while melaena may be replaced by total absence of faeces
- stance may be persistently abnormal after 24 hours, animal adopting rocking-horse position, or may lie down and groan
- site is usually distal jejunum, or rarely jejunoileal junction with invaginated section (intussusceptum) passing into caecum or into proximal colon

Condition may last five to eight days, with slow deterioration and death from metabolic effects of total obstruction in which plasma chloride progressively falls, with haemoconcentration and dehydration.

Diagnosis
Diagnosis depends on rectal palpation of several distended small bowel loops, about 5 cm diameter, or possibly a firm, painful and slightly mobile, fist-shaped mass relatively low on right side or just cranial to pelvic inlet. In

calf bilateral abdominal palpation may suggest a firm irregular abdominal mass. Mass may be out of reach and diagnosis then depends on right-sided exploratory laparotomy. However, severely distended small bowel on rectal palpation or on ultrasound may be a case of small intestinal ileus.

Differential diagnosis: intestinal volvulus, mesenteric torsion. Both have rapid clinical course, and distention of lower right flank with splashing sounds on auscultation.

Treatment

It is alleged that some cases recover spontaneously after sloughing the intus-susceptum, but this has never been seen by the authors.

- i.v. fluids e.g. hypertonic or isotonic saline
- right flank laparotomy under paravertebral analgesia (see Section 1.8, p. 23) and topical analgesia of affected bowel segment and mesentery, possibly also systemic analgesic; alternatively under GA
- standing surgery preferable except in calf < 12 months
- exteriorise affected bowel, and attempt manual reduction in early case
- in case of intestinal wall devitalisation, and where manual reduction is impossible, isolate with clamps, resect bowel segment and mesentery and perform end-to-end or less optimal side-to-side anastomosis
- note that traction on mesenteric root is very painful and may cause animal to collapse, therefore first infiltrate lignocaine into affected segment of mesentery
- suture technique should avoid production of bowel stenosis: single layers of Cushing pattern, interrupted once, is suitable. Some surgeons may oversew with Lembert or Cushing suture (PDS 2 metric with swaged-on needle)
- manage differing pre- and post-stenotic luminal diameters by 45–60° angled incision line in (smaller) post-stenotic bowel
- initial single sutures in the anti-mesenteric and mesenteric borders facilitate manipulation
- closure of mesenteric defect is essential to prevent possible herniation
- preferred material is fine absorbable suture (e.g. 7 metric Softgut® (Davis & Geck)) on 45 mm 3/8 circle round-bodied needle or 3.5 metric PGA
- leakage at suture line is rarely a problem
- maintain strictly aseptic procedure, otherwise massive local peritonitis may result in multiple bowel adhesions
- wash visceral peritoneal surface of bowel with copious volume of sterile physiological saline before closing the abdominal incision
- aftercare should comprise antimicrobials for five to seven days, hay and laxative feeds (e.g. bran) for one week

Successful surgery is evident in passage of loose dark faeces 24–48 hours later.

Caecal invagination is a specific entity seen predominantly in younger calves. Often reducible manually, they often recur, so amputation is preferable (p. 118).

3.11 Other forms of intestinal obstruction

Intestinal obstruction is occasionally caused by other abdominal abnormalities including:

- large pedunculated fatty masses (lipomata)
- large intra-mesenteric areas of fat necrosis
- adventitious fibrous bands
- scrotal hernia, volvulus and incarceration in traumatised vas deferens

Incarceration in traumatised vas deferens ('gut-tie')

Introduction

Obstruction, rarely strangulation, may follow passage of bowel through tear of peritoneum between vas deferens and abdominal wall, following castration procedure in which excessive traction on, and recoil of, spermatic cord results in adhesion of cord or peritoneal fold around bowel ('gut-tie'). Jejunum is usually involved and condition develops slowly with signs related to gradual lumenal occlusion (see Figure 3.19).

Signs

- anorexia, dullness, reduced passage of faeces and distention of flank
- ballottement of flanks and palpation inconclusive
- rectal palpation often permits easy diagnosis by recognition of distended small intestine and one or more abnormal cord-like structures near inguinal ring (see Figure 3.19)
- diagnosis depends on exploratory laparotomy following suggestive history and signs
- problem is usually located near internal inguinal ring and (due to anatomical distribution of small intestine) on right side

Treatment

- gentle rectal traction on adhesed spermatic cord stump is fairly simple to perform and may lead to rapid recovery (90% success) but can be hazardous and not recommended for inexperienced persons who should appreciate the risk of tearing the bowel wall
- perform right flank laparotomy in standing or left laterally recumbent animal
- section or resect the adhesed spermatic cord or vas deferens with scissors using blind palpation

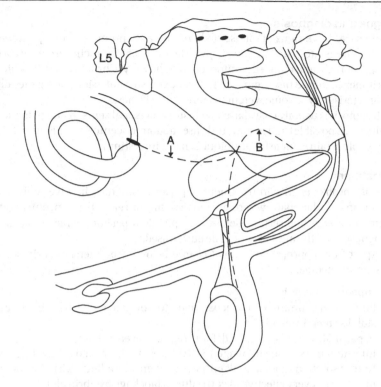

Figure 3.19 'Gut-tie' involving recoiled stump of ductus (vas) deferens adhesing around and occluding lumen of small intestine, resulting in bowel obstruction (compare with Figure 1.11).
A. abnormal stump of ductus (vas) deferens; B. normal position of ductus (vas) deferens.

- exteriorise bowel and check for viability
- resection and anastomosis required in exceptional cases
- routine closure of flank laparotomy incision (see Section 3.3 pp. 86–87).
- post-operative systemic antibiotics for three days, especially if bowel resection was performed

3.12 Peritonitis

Introduction

Peritonitis is usually secondary to a diffuse or localised primary condition. Causes may be perforation of an abomasal ulcer, rupture of a reticular wall or hepatic abscess, reticular perforation of a foreign body, infection following uterine rupture, or the introduction of infection at caesarean section. Some cases follow a breakdown of surgical asepsis.

Signs and diagnosis

Early cases have signs of diffuse abdominal pain and may grunt spontaneously. The acute reaction causes pyrexia (to 40.5°C), tachycardia, arched back, anorexia and reduced ruminoreticular activity. Chronic cases, in which peritoneal exudate has organised to form extensive adhesions, are generally characterised by chronic weight loss and unthriftiness.

Diagnosis is usually easy, based on history, classical signs, rectal palpation (adhesions possible) and in doubtful cases abdominocentesis (see Figure 3.23 – possibly retain sample for antibiotic sensitivity testing).

Treatment

Specific problems arise in treatment of peritonitis, which involves infection in a transcellular space where antibiotics cannot reach the concentrations found in tissues and serum. Generalised purulent peritonitis has a hopeless prognosis, and the animal should be euthanised.

Apart from appropriate antibiotics (see below), treatment in early acute cases may include:

- supportive i.v. fluids
- flunixin meglumine or corticosteroids to counter endotoxic shock and stabilise membranes
- heparin 5000 units, i.m., b.i.d. for three days in early cases
- intermittent peritoneal lavage (5–10 litres, t.i.d. or q.i.d.) with lactated Ringer solution (dorsal flank entry port, ventral midline exit). Peritoneal lavage is not very effective in cattle due to blockage by fibrin clots.

Drugs of choice include:

- tetracyclines, e.g. oxytetracycline (22 mg/kg daily)
- sulphonamides (sulphadimidine, sulphadiazine, or triple sulphas).

See Section 1.12, p. 47, Table 1.15 for extra-label drug use and withdrawal times.

3.13 Umbilical hernia and abscess

Introduction

Umbilical herniation is a very common surgical condition in the Holstein and other cattle breeds. It may be inherited by a dominant character with incomplete penetrance, or be conditioned by environmental factors. It is unlikely to be sex linked.

Complication of herniation is frequently coexistent with umbilical abscessation. Sometimes abscess may be involved in primary aetiology. Surgery may be contra-indicated in large simple (i.e. non-infected) umbilical herniae of animals intended as breeding stock (e.g. bulls), because evidence suggests the condition is inherited (see Section 1.16, pp. 52–53).

Signs

An exceptionally large umbilical hernia is evident at birth, but the majority are first noticed a few weeks later. The peritoneum-lined hernial sac may measure 3–12 cm diameter. Corresponding hernial ring is typically about 1–7 cm long and 1–3 cm wide.

Contents of hernial sac are peritoneal fluid, greater omentum, and in larger cases, the abomasum. Small or large intestine is sometimes involved.

Diagnosis

Diagnosis is based on the history, palpation of the swelling and the adjacent ventral abdominal wall for signs of intra-abdominal involvement. Pain on palpation is suspicious of a septic process (see Figure 3.20) or incarceration. Ultrasound investigation may be considered to define the contents of an umbilical swelling and intra-abdominal involvement.

Indications for surgery

Calves under four weeks old should only be operated as an emergency, since stress of anaesthesia may be critical to survival, and abscess capsule may not be thick enough for safe resection.

Otherwise, indications include:

- irreducible (incarcerated or strangulated) hernial contents irrespective of age, size and intended use of calf
- increasing hernial size

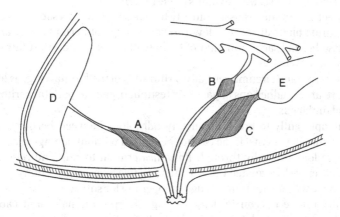

Figure 3.20 Three sites of umbilical infection with intra-abdominal involvement. A. umbilical vein (purulent omphalophlebitis); B. umbilical artery (purulent omphaloarteritis); C. urachus (purulent urachitis); D. liver; E. bladder.

- calves aged three to six months with hernia still present, possibly enlarging, since spontaneous resolution is now unlikely

Pre-operative complications:

- an encapsulated abscess makes surgery more awkward and potentially hazardous, but contamination of wound is not inevitable
- treat discharging umbilical sinus by repeated local irrigation and débridement, and possibly systemic antibiotics for three to five days. If still not resolved, discharging umbilical abscess cavity should be packed with swabs and overlying skin tightly sutured before starting surgery

Surgical technique

- reduce ruminal volume in older calves by 24 hours' starvation to reduce post-op pressure on surgical wound, also to reduce degree of ruminal tympany during surgery, both during GA and LA
- obtain deep sedation and perform local analgesic infiltration of area with or without anterior epidural analgesia, or use GA (see Section 1.9, pp. 36–39)
- place calf in dorsal recumbency, preferably raised from ground, and positioned with straw bales laterally, and with legs fixed cranially and caudally remote from surgical field
- in male calf irrigate and pack preputial cavity
- clip extensive area of ventral abdominal wall, scrub and disinfect three times
- ensure availability of sterile prosthetic mesh material for hernias where ring exceeds 10 cm diameter (see below)
- make elliptical skin incision around hernial base, continue along midline well cranial and caudal to limits of hernial ring
- dissect subcutaneous tissue bluntly to expose the hernial sac
- continue blunt dissection down to reveal edge of hernial ring, carefully incise hernial sac at junction of body wall and sac and insert finger into abdominal cavity
- resect sac, and circumferentially a thin strip of the hernial ring, as long as there are no adhesions of gastro-intestinal organs to parietal peritoneum and umbilicus
- attempt gently to break down any adhesions between hernial sac and abdominal contents. If sac cannot be incised without damaging contents, incise longitudinally through *linea alba* cranial to ring and remove sac together with herniated viscera after any necessary enterectomy
- bring together longitudinal edges of opening for suturing
- avoid undue tension by lengthening the ring cranially and caudally, converting the oval shape into a long ellipse
- if ring closure is likely to result in excessive suture tension, make longitudinal incision through external sheath of the rectus sheath, about

3 cm lateral to left and right of midline. Incision should not extend into longitudinal muscle fibres or the internal rectus sheath
- close body defect wall by simple interrupted sutures of absorbable material such as polyglactin 910, PGA or PDS starting at commissures of the wound
- use a near-far-far-near pattern in large hernias
- if approximation for tying knots is difficult, preplace sutures and secure ends loosely with haemostatic forceps, and then use steady traction on all the sutures finally to close the ring
- internal hernial sac may alternatively be reduced into abdomen and edges of ring apposed in same manner but without penetrating peritoneum (closed herniorraphy), but recurrence common
- ensure sutures are well covered by subcutaneous tissues closed by PDS 5 metric in continuous pattern. It is essential to bury the deep suture layer and to avoid leaving potential dead space
- appose the skin edges by vertical mattress sutures (monofilament nylon)
- eliminate dead space by resecting excessive skin tissue
- give systemic antibiotics for three to five days
- clean skin wound with warm dilute povidone-iodine solution after 24 hours, or preferably abdominal wrap for 24 hours confining calf in box for one to two weeks
- give only water and a little concentrate for the first two days, after which normal diet is resumed

Vital points in surgical procedure include:

- do not penetrate any encapsulated infection (e.g. umbilical abscess)
- aseptic technique
- careful haemostasis
- gentle handling of relatively friable tissues

Prosthetic material repair
Prosthetic repair of umbilical hernias and other abdominal wall defects is seldom necessary in cattle. Indications include large hernias, cases in which repair has been unsuccessfully attempted by simple closure, and incisional hernias following abomasopexy or caesarean section (see Figure 3.21).
Suitable materials for mesh include:

- woven plastic or polypropylene mesh – strong, inert, easily handled, and cheap, e.g. Mersilene® (Ethicon), Marlex® (Dowd Inc., Providence, RI, USA), Proxplast® (Goshen), preferably inserted doubled or absorbable Vicryl® (Ethicon)

Rarely used are stainless steel gauze (very strong, inert, less easily handled and expensive), and tantalum (Fansteel Metals, Chicago) which has properties as for plastic or polypropylene, but is also expensive.

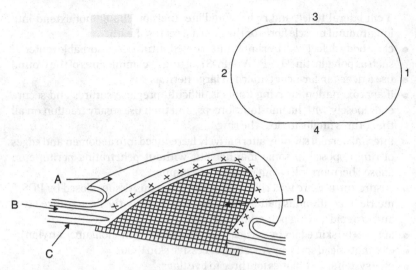

Figure 3.21 Mesh implant in large umbilical hernia.
A. skin and subcutaneous tissues; B. *linea alba* and internal rectus sheath;
C. peritoneum (sac dissected away); D. mesh sutured with 1 cm overlap onto
peritoneum and internal rectus sheath/*linea alba*; (inset shows suggested order of
insertion, 1 being cranial).

Technique

It is frequently impossible to avoid inserting the material into the abdominal
cavity, although ideally the internal hernial ring and parietal peritoneum
should be left intact, the hernial sac inverted, and the mesh should be buried
underneath the parietal peritoneum.

- ensure that the size of mesh prepared is slightly larger in area than the
  defect
- suture initially to four equidistant points of circumference e.g. caudal,
  cranial, left lateral, right lateral. Normally distal contact surface will be
  greater omentum
- trim to precise size
- place interrupted simple or vertical mattress pattern sutures into firm
  fibrous tissue of hernial ring (see Figure 3.21)
- bury mesh with layer of connective tissue. Mesh must not lie
  subcutaneously
- avoid any residual dead space by resection of excessive skin before insertion of interrupted vertical mattress skin sutures

Complications of umbilical hernia repair

- seroma formation and eventually infection of this fluid with abscessation
- haematoma: should be left untreated but if subcutaneous tissues then become infected, drainage must be provided at once and the cavity flushed twice daily (with povidone-iodine), also start systemic antibiotics
- breakdown of hernial repair (dehiscence) with prolapse of omentum to occupy subcutaneous space: early re-operation imperative to avoid incarceration, adhesions and early development of diffuse peritonitis

Treatment of encapsulated umbilical abscessation by surgery

- extra-capsular dissection is essential to avoid gross contamination and peritonitis
- at early stage any tract should be followed into abdominal cavity by palpation and/or ultrasonography to establish direction, i.e. cranially towards liver if umbilical vein (septic thrombophlebitis) or caudally towards bladder vertex (septic urachus, or septic arteritis) (see Figure 3.20)
- careful exploration with a sterile probe is often helpful
- paramedian laparotomy at level of umbilicus permits inspection and dissection of such infected tracts

Infection of the umbilical vein is serious, as sepsis may extend into the liver, permitting haematogenous spread to lungs, joints ('joint ill') and other organs. Resection is then contra-indicated. If no spread has occurred, and the vein is involved in septic thrombophlebitis, marsupialisation through the ventral abdominal wall under GA may be attempted in valuable stock.

In most cases of septic thrombrophlebitis and septic urachitis, resection is simple under GA. Surgical excision of the infected urachus, arteries or vein should be complete. The stumps of healthy tissue can, at the surgeon's discretion, be oversewn with greater omentum. Sometimes small area of bladder wall continuous with pervious urachus is resected and the opening closed by continuous inversion suture.

Post-operative treatment: systemic antimicrobial therapy for five days.

3.14 Alimentary conditions involving neoplasia

Alimentary tract neoplasms are, with the exception below, uncommon. Some are seen in the oral cavity (fibroma, sarcoma) requiring differential diagnosis from actinobacillosis and actinomycosis. Intestinal neoplasms have occasionally been incriminated in the pathogenesis of intussusception, and are then amenable to removal via bowel resection and anastomosis. Lipomata are sometimes the cause of vague indigestion and weight loss in adult cattle, especially the Channel Island breeds, and are rarely treatable.

Squamous cell carcinoma

Squamous cell carcinoma (SCC), has the highest incidence of any cancer in the world in certain upland areas and, since alimentary tract signs may be seen, this problem is discussed briefly. SCC develops in any part of the alimentary tract (oropharynx, oesophagus, oesophageal groove, rumen) as a proliferative, scirrhous, and often ulcerating series of masses, sometimes preceded by squamous papillomata.

Occurrence is exclusively in upland areas where older cattle (exceeding eight years, usually beef types) have had prolonged exposure for several years to bracken (*Pteridium aquilinum*). The toxic factor is ptaquiloside. There is a history of acute bracken poisoning in about 50% of cases of SCC.

Its relationship to papilloma virus, which produces non-infiltrating sessile warts, is not yet precisely established. About one third of affected cattle have lesions of enzootic haematuria.

Clinical signs
These may have four forms:

- oropharyngeal – loss of condition, drooling of saliva, coughing, halitosis, enlarged submandibular lymph nodes, nasal discharge containing ingesta, and diarrhoea. A large fungating mass may involve the tongue base, pharynx and palate, or several smaller lesions may exist
- oesophageal – progressive weight loss for one to three months, cud dropping, palpable oesophageal mass, mild halitosis, drooling saliva, coughing, gurgling sounds from oesophagus, diarrhoea, resistance to passage of stomach tube and oropharyngeal papillomata
- chronic ruminal tympany – mild, or less commonly relatively sudden and severe onset with loss of condition for one to six months, profuse diarrhoea, possible resistance to passage of stomach tube due to papillomata in oropharynx
- wasting diarrhoea – loss of condition and chronic diarrhoea for one to nine months, initially profuse and watery, later leaving fibrous mass in ruminoreticulum possibly also oropharyngeal papillomata

Diagnosis
Careful inspection is made of oropharynx with mouth gag (Drinkwater pattern), torch and manual exploration. Endoscopy of oesophagus if available.

Some cases with clinical signs, including chronic tympany referable to ruminoreticulum, undergo exploratory laparotomy (no significant findings) and, more usefully, rumenotomy when one or more large fungating and ulcerating masses up to 12 cm diameter may be detected in or near the oesophageal groove and cardia.

Complete removal of ruminoreticular lesions with resolution of the clinical signs is impossible due to extensive mural infiltration. Biopsy material may be taken for diagnostic pathology. Such cases are almost invariably found retrospectively to have lesions in the oropharynx.

The prognosis is hopeless and affected cattle should be slaughtered.

3.15 Vagal indigestion (Hoflund syndrome)

Introduction
Vagal (vagus) indigestion is a chronic ruminoreticular condition of increasing abdominal distension and low-grade ruminoreticular activity, thought to be associated with dysfunction of vagal nerve branches supplying the forestomachs. Dysfunction involves hyper- or hypomotility, and often results in a secondary abomasal tympany.

Anatomy
The left and right vagus nerves (see Figure 3.22) form dorsal and ventral oesophageal trunks and supply direct branches to the ruminoreticular wall, including the sulcus and reticulo-omasal orifice, omasum and abomasum. Section of both trunks completely abolishes motor activity of the forestomachs. Section of the dorsal branch alone results in almost complete, but not inevitably permanent, paralysis of the rumen, with lesser effects on the reticulum. The effects of section of the ventral branch are less predictable and range from little to almost complete forestomach paralysis.

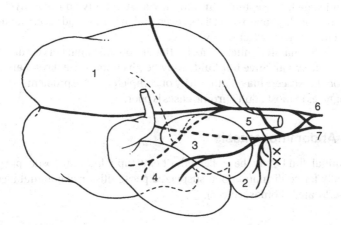

Figure 3.22 Vagal trunk innervation of bovine stomachs, viewed from right side. 1. dorsal sac or rumen; 2. reticulum; 3. omasum; 4. abomasum; 5. cardia; 6 & 7 dorsal and ventral trunks of vagus lying alongside oesophagus at cardia.
Note that abscessation in reticular wall (x) is liable to interfere with innervation, particularly of the omentum and abomasum. Dorsal vagal trunk (6) primarily innervates rumen. (modified from Dyce & Wensing, 1971.)

Clinical signs

Signs develop following alleged injury to the vagal nerves either in the thoracic mediastinum or in the cranial abdominal cavity, commonly due to extensive peritonitis secondary to traumatic reticulitis.

- movement of ingesta from rumenoreticulum into the omasum and abomasum is grossly disturbed due to a functional stenosis and hypomotility of the omasum
- bradycardia often present (< 60/min)
- usually adult cows with a history of weight loss and increasing abdominal distension often around pasturition
- frequently history of an episode of acute traumatic reticulitis
- viewed caudally, animal has a 'ten-to-four' or 'papple' (pear right, apple left) distension, i.e. upper left flank and lower right flank
- ruminal distension possibly associated with hypomotility or atony, reduced feed intake, and scanty faeces. Other cattle show hypermotility but abnormal rumen contents
- careful deep palpation through left flank reveals the ruminal contents to be completely mixed and not triple-layered (gas/firm solid material/fluid)

Treatment

Exploratory laparotomy and rumenotomy are indicated to check abdominal cavity between cranial surface of reticulum and diaphragm. Rumenotomy may rarely reveal lesions of actinobacillosis, which is amenable to treatment: sodium iodide i.v. streptomycin and dihydrostreptomycin (Devomycin D®, Norbrook), on days one, three, five, seven and nine or broad spectrum antibiotics (tetracyclines) systemically.

Cases with massive adhesion formation involving vagal nerves: any treatment is purely palliative but fluids may be given for some days. Lancing of perireticular abscess may temporarily or completely solve problem.

Prognosis in most adult chronic cases is poor.

3.16 Abdominocentesis

Abdominal fluid may be collected ('belly tap') for diagnostic purposes, generally for confirmation of a suspected peritonitis or abdominal bleeding (e.g. perforated abomasal ulcer).

Technique

- clip and surgical scrub (diluted povidone-iodine) right ventral abdominal wall cranial to umbilicus over most pendulous part (cranial quadrant) or medial to the fold of the flank and 'milk vein' (caudal quadrant), in each case 5 cm from midline (see Figure 3.23)

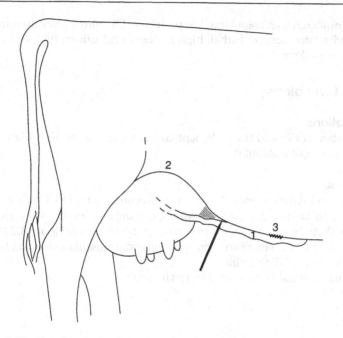

Figure 3.23   Possible site for abdominocentesis on right side of abdominal wall in angle between right abdominal ('milk') vein (1) and stifle fold (2). Arrow shows site of needle puncture; (3) shows level of umbilicus.

- tail restraint with animal in crush
- insert 16 gauge 3.7–5 cm needle through skin, and slowly advance to 'pop' through fascia and parietal peritoneum
- needle tip is palpably free in abdominal cavity
- if no fluid drips, first rotate needle and slightly change angle
- attach 5 ml sterile syringe and slowly withdraw plunger (rarely successful!)
- normal fluid is pale yellow (volume < 5 ml, odourless)
- if abdominal viscus such as omental fat is entered, another site should be selected with new needle

Discussion
Fluid may be collected in EDTA tubes for a total white blood cell count, or sterile tubes for culture. Visual inspection should alone differentiate conditions such as diffuse peritonitis, haemoperitoneum and uroperitoneum from normal fluid.

Transudate: clear, colourless, low protein (< 2.5 g/litre), low cell count
Exudate: discoloured, turbid, high protein (> 2.5 g/litre) high cell count,
frothy on shaking

3.17 Liver biopsy

Indications
Estimation of Cu, and trace element concentration; diagnosis of fatty liver
and other hepatic pathology.

Technique
- clip and disinfect area 15 × 15 cm, centred on 11th (10th in very
  long-backed cattle) right intercostal space and 20 cm ventral to vertebrae.
  Check site by percussion for area of hepatic dullness (see Figure 3.24)
- produce local analgesia of skin and intercostal musculature by infiltration
  of 5–10 ml 2% lignocaine
- make 1 cm stab incision in skin and musculature

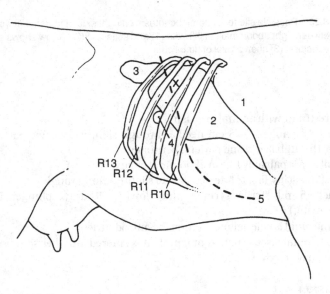

Figure 3.24   Diagram of right side of abdominal wall of cow, showing site of hepatic
dullness. Cranial boundary is usually around rib 9. In severe hepatomegaly caudal
border may be palpable behind last rib. Site for hepatic biopsy is about one third of
distance down rib cage. (From Smart & Northcote, 1985.)
1. lung; 2. liver; 3. right kidney; 4. gall bladder; 5. phrenico-costal line; X site of liver
biopsy.

- insert trocar and cannula (20 cm long, 6 mm external diameter, see Appendix 3 for manufacturers) through incision, through intercostal muscle
- perforate parietal peritoneum (palpable sensation, also pain reaction likely in animal) to contact liver surface
- withdraw trocar and advance cannula at angle of 70° to horizontal and 20° cranially (i.e. slightly downwards and forwards, aiming towards left elbow) using slightly rotating action
- if necessary, partly withdraw cannula and repeat in slightly changed direction: characteristic soft grinding sensation is appreciable on passage through liver
- attach adapter and syringe (tight fit essential), and using continuous negative pressure, twist and then withdraw cannula and contained tissue
- expel tissue (typical specimen 4 cm × 4 mm diameter) onto dry gauze swab by positive pressure, or reinsertion of trocar
- dress skin wound with dry antibiotic powder, suture unnecessary. Procedure may be safely repeated at weekly intervals. Manufacturer of biopsy instrument is given in Appendix 3, pp. 262–265.

Complications
- accidental entry into hepatic vessel – immediate bleeding from cannula. Avoid by stopping advance of cannula should any firm structure (namely perivascular fibrous tissue) be encountered, and changing direction slightly
- accidental entry into hepatic abscess with gross peritonitis
- localised peritonitis – dirty technique
- wound infection – dirty technique

3.18 Anal and rectal atresia

Introduction
Anal and rectal atresia (imperforate anus) in the calf are rare, anal atresia being more frequent. Inheritance of this lethal defect in cattle is not established. Other defects e.g. taillessness and spinal dysraphia may co-exist.

Diagnosis
Usually made at two to three days old unless stockman has made meticulous, neonatal examination. Absence of faeces draws attention to calf which may have slightly distended abdomen.

Perineum has a scar indicative of anal orifice. In anal atresia scar may overlie a slight bulge of the subcutaneous tissues, and becomes more pronounced on increased intra-abdominal pressure, applied by pushing on the flanks or by spontaneous tenesmus. Absence of such a bulge suggests that rectal atresia may also be present.

Investigation of differential diagnosis between atresia involving anus alone and both anus and caudal rectum depends on surgical exploration.

Surgery

- operate as soon as possible under caudal epidural analgesia (1 ml 2% lignocaine plain)
- cleanse and clip area 10 cm diameter around anus
- remove 1 cm diameter circle of skin over anal scar
- retract skin edges with Allis forceps held by assistant
- in anal atresia a distended blind-ended rectum is easily located by digital exploration in pelvic midline
- attempt to suture rectal wall to skin at this stage
- otherwise gently break down surrounding connective tissue and attempt to exteriorise the caudal portion of rectum
- place four stay sutures dorsally, ventrally and bilaterally into rectum to maintain in position and then incise this vertically for 1–2 cm; meconium will spurt from lumen
- suture rectal margin to skin in simple interrupted sutures of 4 metric chromic catgut, starting with two dorsal sutures at eleven o'clock and one o'clock positions, followed by two ventrally at seven o'clock and five o'clock
- add additional sutures laterally
- avoid as far as possible contamination of subcutis and, more important, the pelvic cavity
- remove extra-rectal meconium with damp swabs and do not irrigate wound which could flush infection cranially
- inject systemic antibiotics (five days)
- maintain a lumen, minimum 2 cm diameter, which may require dilatation several weeks later as initial healing results in localised fibrosis
- milk diet for two weeks
- do not use for breeding

Rectal atresia

Treatment

Calves with additional atresia involving the rectum may prove difficult to assess, and impossible to correct without the creation of a low flank caecal fistula (preternatal anus) which, though possible experimentally, cannot be justified on economic, practical and animal welfare grounds. Cicatricial stricture is a common post-operative result.

Slight rectal atresia, with the rectum terminating 2 cm cranial to the anus, is treated by careful blunt dissection dorsally involving the mesorectum; suture to skin as for anal atresia.

Unfortunately in many cases the integrity of the blood supply is seriously impaired by inadvertent tears and stretching of the mesorectum, causing mural necrosis followed by rupture of the rectal wall and fatal faecal peritonitis extending from the pelvic cavity into the abdomen. Euthanasia is therefore advisable in cases of anal and rectal atresia which involve absence of at least 3 cm of terminal rectum.

3.19 Rectal prolapse

Introduction
Rectal prolapse seen in young calves, yearling cattle and rarely adults may be:

- incomplete – prolapse of mucosal layer only, with local oedema
- complete – total eversion of caudal rectum with serosal rectal surfaces in contact

Aetiology and signs
- prime sign is marked tenesmus, usually as a result of severe localised pain
- severe enteritis involving passage of sloughed epithelial debris and blood, as in severe acute salmonellosis or coccidiosis
- sudden high protein intake with diarrhoea
- rarely due to other causes, e.g. urolithiasis (severe straining), severe ruminal tympany, high oestrogen intake (causing relaxation of ischiorectal fossa), following a vaginal prolapse or rabies

Diagnosis
Diagnosis is easily made. Degree of contusion and laceration should be established when cleaning the prolapse after inducing caudal epidural analgesia (see Section 1.8, pp. 27–29).

Treatment
Three forms can be distinguished. All may be performed under epidural anaesthesia (1–2 ml of 2% lignocaine):

(a) Recent incomplete prolapse without mucosal injury:
- replacement and purse-string suture in subcutaneous peri-anal skin
- insert needle ventrally, emerging dorsally to expose minimum length of non-absorbable material (e.g. sterile nylon tape) to possible contamination
- suture should be tied in bow ventrally to permit gradual controlled slackening
- suture should permit adequate passage of faeces but prevent re-prolapse, and in a one-month-old calf should permit entry of two digits

(b) Recent incomplete prolapse with mucosal injury:
- suture tear, or if impossible, perform rectal amputation or sub-mucosal resection (see below)

(c) Complete prolapse:
- attempt replacement if not severely traumatised. Bathing with dilute Epsom salts or tannic acid solution may reduce size of oedematous mass

If replacement is impossible two procedures are available, laborious sub-mucosal resection and amputation.

Submucosal resection
- make two circular incisions around circumference of the rectum, through mucosa to the submucosal tissue. The first incision is at the point where the rectum is reflected on itself, the second is about 1 cm from mucocut-aneous junction
- join two incisions by another dorsal incision at right angles, and longit-udinal in direction
- dissect and remove 'sleeve' of rectal mucosa between the two circular incisions
- effect haemostasis by swab pressure and ligation of large vessels
- appose mucosal edges in row of interrupted simple sutures of 4 metric PDS
- insert purse-string suture as described above

Amputation
Two techniques are available.

Technique 1   Stairstep amputation:
- initially put plastic syringe casing into lumen of rectum and insert cross-pin fixation with two hypodermic needles to stabilise the prolapsed rectum during suturing procedure (see Figure 3.25)
- make circumferential incision cranial to necrotic area, but do not cut inner mucosa and inner submucosa
- create stairstep and amputate 3 cm caudal to initial circumferential incision
- use extra tissue (inner mucosal layer) to reduce tension on the circum-ferential suture
- remove hypodermic needles and syringe casing and insert purse-string suture, as above

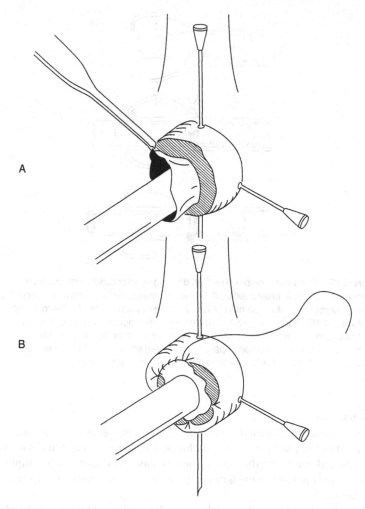

Figure 3.25 Stair-step amputation of the prolapsed rectum A and suture of mucosa B.

Technique 2 Termed 'rectal ring' method (see Figure 3.26):

- take plastic syringe case, open at each end, or proprietary product, and anchor with circumferential monofilament nylon suture at the most proximal part of the prolapse
- blood supply is effectively occluded to distal rectum, which sloughs about 10 days later

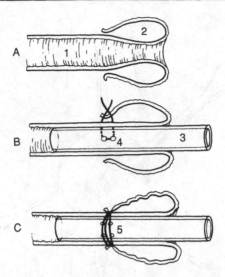

Figure 3.26 Repair of prolapsed rectum utilising syringe case or plastic tubing.
A. lumen of rectum; 2. prolapsed wall. B Sutures are placed through skin-rectal
mucosal junction and through holes (4) in the side of plastic tube (3). Second sutures
are placed at 180° to first suture. C Sutures are pulled tight over skin as tube is
inserted appropriately within rectal lumen. Sutures are then tied around the
circumference to occlude blood supply to prolapsed section (5). Prolapsed rectum
and tube drop off some days later as a result of ischaemic necrosis.

Discussion

Careful check must be made at frequent intervals, following technique 2, to
ensure that the plastic case has not become dislodged, and that defaecation
can proceed normally through lumen of case. The method is simple but
messy, and fails if the casing is dislodged for example by contact with pen wall
or other cattle.

Post-operative tenesmus is delayed if the epidural block is made with a
xylazine-lignocaine mixture (see Section 1.7, p. 29) or a longer acting analgesic drug (e.g. Bupivacaine®).

Complications

- immediate excessive stenosis – resuture placing larger diameter hollow
  casing into lumen
- excessive haemorrhage – oversew vessel including full thickness of wall
- severe continuous postoperative tenesmus – repeat long-acting epidural
  block, produce pneumoperitoneum (insufflating through needle placed
  in left paralumbar fossa and attached to Higginson's syringe), slacken
  purse-string suture

- anal stricture due to excessive fibrosis – incise anus dorsally and ventrally through depth of fibrous tissue, and suture cranial commissure to caudal commissure of wound

Prophylaxis involves attention to the underlying causes (e.g. diet) for the initial development of the rectal prolapse, especially important in cases where there are several affected individuals.

CHAPTER 4

Female urinogenital surgery

4.1 Caesarean section (hysterotomy)

Indications
- excessive fetal size (immaturity of dam, double muscling, genetic mis-matching, and prolonged gestation)
- fetal deformity (e.g. *schistosoma reflexus*)
- relative or absolute narrowness of pelvic canal (immaturity of dam, traumatic pelvic deformity)
- fetal malpresentation or posture
- irreducible uterine torsion, uterine rupture, non or incomplete dilatation of cervical os
- atresia or hypoplasia of maternal vagina or vulva
- certain valuable pedigree breeding programmes where safe delivery of a viable fetus is paramount, and where management precludes the risks associated with natural delivery

Until recently hydroallantois and hydroamnion were further indications for two-stage caesarean section (day one: slow drainage of uterine fluids; day two: caesarean section). Such cases today have a better prognosis if treated before onset of recumbency with corticosteroids or prostaglandins, followed several days later by an i.v. oxytocin drip in refractory cases.

Contra-indications
- cattle in very poor bodily condition (cachectic)
- emphysematous fetus
- most cows with uterine infection

Caesarean section may still be preferable to embryotomy (fetotomy) in cases of general debility and prolonged dystocia despite the presence of dead fetus.

Advantages of caesarean section over embryotomy include:

- potential fetal survival
- usually faster and safer procedure
- feasibility where embryotomy would be impossible (cervical non-dilatation)

Surgical technique: Flank

Xylazine premedication is contra-indicated due to induced increase of myometrial tone. If permitted a uterine relaxant (e.g. clenbuterol HCl 300 µg) should be given i.m. or slowly i.v. to facilitate rotation and partial exteriorisation of the uterus.

Operate if possible on standing cow or heifer under lumbar paravertebral block (T13, L1–3, see Section 1.8, p. 23), but weak debilitated and ataxic cattle should be cast before surgery, and in such cases cranial epidural block is a feasible alternative analgesic method (60–80 ml 2% lignocaine). Another possibility is a 30 ml caudal epidural block and inverted '7' or 'L' flank analgesia (see p. 26); tie tail to hind leg.

Left flank site is preferred to right flank unless specific indication for right side exists (e.g. over-sized fetus in right flank, grossly distended rumen). On right side small intestinal loops are more liable to prolapse through wound to become traumatised and infected.

- give caudal epidural block (e.g. 5 ml 2% lignocaine) to any cow which is straining considerably, as tenesmus hampers precise incision of uterus, and can even provoke ruminal wall prolapse through flank incision
- clip, scrub and disinfect entire paralumbar fossa (last rib to hip) and apply sterile drapes
- make 30–35 cm vertical incision in middle or caudal third of left paralumbar fossa (see Figure 3.6(4) and effect careful haemostasis of flank vessels
- insert hand into abdomen pushing rumen forward and feeling ventrally and caudally
- make rapid assessment of fetal position and condition of uterine wall
- attempt to bring greater curvature of gravid horn towards abdominal incision by always grasping uterine wall over protruding part of fetus (e.g. limb, hock in anterior presentation)
- attempt to exteriorise greater curvature of gravid horn
- note that, unless there is severe intra-uterine infection (e.g. grossly emphysematous fetus), entry of uterine fluid to contaminate abdominal cavity is rarely hazardous
- grasp fetal leg (e.g. digits or point of hock) through uterine wall and maintain firmly in flank section
- incise uterine wall (see Figure 4.1) along greater curvature adjacent to the limb and towards the tip of the horn with scalpel blade or finger embryotomy (fetotomy) knife starting below digits and extending to hock (or carpus in forelimb, if in posterior presentation)

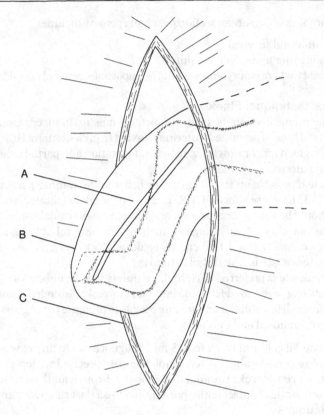

Figure 4.1 Uterine incision (greater curvature) over right hind metatarsus and foot, having partially exteriorised fetus.
A. uterine incision; B. exteriorised horn; C. left flank incision.

- avoid incising maternal caruncles (see Figure 4.1)
- extend incision very carefully caudally until the limb can be exteriorised for application of obstetric chain or rope
- instruct assistant to maintain very gentle traction on rope/chain sufficient to maintain uterine wall in flank incision
- lengthen uterine incision to permit entry of hand into uterus to locate second limb, which is similarly exteriorised and a rope/chain applied
- manipulate head best by a thumb and finger grip in each orbit
- if very large fetus or uterine horn tip cannot be brought to flank wound for incision under direct vision, make blind incision over fetal extremity, which is then grasped and brought to flank in similar manner
- ensure that fetal traction is applied gently and in appropriate direction, usually initially upwards, and lengthen uterine incision, if required, with knife to avoid any tearing of uterine wall

- practise careful and slow fetal manipulation during extraction especially in cases of *schistosoma reflexus*, muscle contracture and emphysematous calves
- in case of gross fetal oversize or ankylosis the skin incision may, occasionally, require enlargement to 40 cm
- permit umbilical cord to rupture naturally
- after delivery hold uterine incision in flank wound and remove any loose protruding portions of placenta, leaving remainder *in situ*
- do not attempt to separate placenta from maternal caruncles
- with little or no assistance available, non-crushing uterine clamps (vulsellum forceps) can be used to hold uterus in position
- check for a second fetus in all cases
- intra-uterine medication is unnecessary
- while fetus is being revived and umbilical cord is checked, undertake uterine repair rapidly
- wash uterine wall with saline if needed
- close uterus with continuous Cushing suture, followed by continuous Lembert, or a modified Cushing (Utrecht uterine suture with buried knots)
- suture of uterine wall: start at caudal ventral commissure of wound if a single layer closure is intended or cranially if two layers are to be inserted. Suture material is either 5 or 6 metric PGA, polyglactin or 7 metric chromic catgut (see Figure 4.2)
- in some cases uterine contraction, tone and turgidity permit only simple apposition as sutures tear out when inversion is attempted

Evacuation of fetal and other contaminating fluids from abdominal cavity is usually unnecessary. In case of grossly infected fluids, removal must be attempted by swabs and aspiration. Give intra-abdominal antibiotic or parenteral medication as required. Flank wound is closed in routine manner. Inject oxytocin (50 iu) parenterally to promote uterine contraction.

Post-operative care
Continue parenteral antibiotics for five days especially if a dead calf was delivered, as prophylaxis against infection from retained placenta. Assess patients in severe shock and recumbency by following parameters: general appearance, rectal temperature, heart rate and character, colour of visible membranes, capillary refill time, and willingness to attempt to stand (see p. 41).

In severe cases not only will flunixin meglumine and massive antibiotic medication be required, but such animals also need large volumes of intravenous fluids (e.g. 25 litres).

The calf should be given maternal colostrum as soon as possible by bottle (teat), or oesophageal feeder. The dam should be encouraged to stand to permit suckling as soon as possible.

Placenta is usually released and discharged within 24 hours of surgery, and is a good prognostic sign. Cases with persistent infected discharge at this

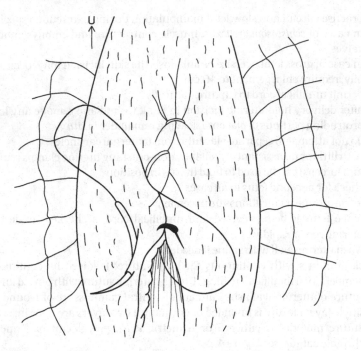

Figure 4.2 Utrecht uterine closure method with knot burial. Needle is inserted at slight angle towards incision and does not penetrate uterine lumen. Sutures are placed sufficiently close to prevent leakage of uterine fluid. Care is taken to avoid placenta.

time should receive systemic antibiotics. Farmer should check rectal temperature and recall veterinarian if cow is febrile.

Healing of the flank wound may occur by secondary intention as a result of intra-operative contamination, and excessive blood and fluid accumulation between suture layers.

Death rate following caesarean section is low (approximately 10%, even lower if cows with poor prognosis are not operated), and is due to:

- endotoxaemic shock
- chronic severe intra-uterine haemorrhage (via vulva)
- septic metritis and peritonitis

Surgical technique: Midline
Ventral midline is a good surgical approach in young beef heifers and in case of large distended and septic uterus; it requires excellent restraint involving more manpower.

- cast at oblique angle between right lateral and dorsal recumbency and restrain legs
- clip and scrub operative field from 12 cm cranial to umbilicus caudally to udder, and cover body with sterile drape with 30 cm window
- incise skin caudally from 5–7 cm cranial to umbilicus as required
- incise fat, fascia, *linea alba* and peritoneum longitudinally
- push free edge of greater omentum cranially and exteriorise gravid horn by traction on fetal limb
- proceed then as for flank incision. Omentum can be drawn over uterine incision before closing body wall
- suture peritoneum and *linea alba* with simple continuous or interrupted appositional mattress eversion suture of PGA or monofilament nylon (7 metric)
- bury this layer with simple continuous layer of chromic catgut
- suture skin and subcutis with monofilament nylon in interrupted mattress pattern

Discussion of other sites for caesarean section

Numerous other sites have been used, and have major disadvantages and certain advantages:

- an oblique mid-left flank incision (ventrolateral or 'Liverpool approach') may improve access to a large gravid uterus. Start 8–10 cm cranial and vertical to tuber coxae ending just caudal to last rib (see Figure 3.6(5))
- oblique low flank incision, medial to fold of stifle, about 20 cm dorsal to attachment of udder skin (Hannover approach, lateral recumbency) with less difficult manipulation of uterus in cases of marked fetal oversize, it avoids well vascularised musculature of flank; good restraint essential if in lateral recumbency (ropes, straps); wound in unfavourable position if complications develop in healing process (see Figure 3.6(3))
- left or right paramedian incision: advantages and disadvantages as for the preceding approach (e.g. easier fetal removal, but restraint problems likely on farm)

It is claimed, but not proven, that uterine adhesions to abdominal viscera are commonly associated with the exposed suture material, especially the knots. The suggested remedy of buried chromic catgut sutures (see Figure 4.2) proposed by the Utrecht school requires confirmation in a controlled study.

Post-operative fertility

Post-operative fertility following caesarean section is lower than fertility following normal parturition (about 72% compared with 89%). Repeat operation is relatively common, though the indication is rarely the same. Comparative data for large series on fertility following embryotomy and caesarean section is lacking.

4.2 Vaginal and cervical prolapse

Introduction
This condition is typically seen in late gestation or the early post-partum period in fat beef (especially Hereford and Santa Gertrudis) and dairy breeds (Holstein and Channel Island).

The chronic case which starts about the eighth or ninth month of gestation presents quite different problems from the post-parturient form, and salvage after parturition is the best solution, as it will recur in the succeeding gestation.

Predisposing factors
- excessive fat deposition in perivaginal connective tissue
- relaxation of sacrotuberous ligaments due to hormonal influence (endocrine imbalance)
- increased intra-abdominal pressure following greater abdominal size in late pregnancy
- high roughage intake
- severe cold weather and poor conformation (large flaccid vulva)
- severe post-partum tenesmus due to vaginal injury
- inheritance is postulated in some Hereford bloodlines, but not proven

Treatment of pre-parturient chronic case
Caudal epidural analgesia is followed by thorough cleaning and replacement of vagina.

Moderate cases of vaginal prolapse in pregnant cows not near to term (e.g. seven months gestation) are best treated by a modified Caslick's operation to close the dorsal vulvar commissure, which is then cut at parturition to avoid vulvar tears. Severe cases near term can be managed in two ways.

Technique 1 Perivulvar suture using Bühner's method (see Figure 4.3):

- surgical scrub of perivulvar area, and careful cleansing of exposed vagina
- place subcutaneous suture of nylon tape in deep tissues around vulva with long vulvar needle (Gerlach pattern, Arnolds, Jorgensen)
- insert needle, threaded with 45 cm sterile nylon tape about 0.6 cm wide, approximately 3 cm below ventral vulvar commissure and directed dorsally through deep connective tissue, to emerge midway between dorsal commissure of vulva and anus
- leave one end of tape hanging from the lower incision, remove the other end from the needle eye, and withdraw the needle
- re-insert unthreaded needle in similar manner along the other edge of the vulvar lip, to emerge adjacent to the original exit point, rethread and pull tape out ventrally (see Figure 4.3)
- tie tape so that adjustment in tension can easily be made

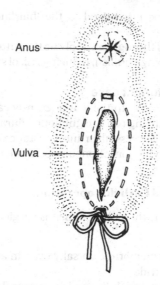

Anus

Vulva

Figure 4.3 Pattern of Bühner suture in vulvar lips. The Gerlach-type needle, threaded with umbilical tape, is inserted below ventral vulvar commissure, and is passed through dense fibrous tissue to emerge above dorsal commissure. It is unthreaded, and needle alone is passed up the other side in similar manner. It is rethreaded, and tape pulled back ventrally. A quick release and adjustable knot is tied. Suture material is only visible at the commissures.

Vulvar lumen should permit easy entry of four fingers. Only about 1 cm length of tape is in contact with vulvar skin dorsally and ventrally. Sutures may be completely buried by two 1 cm long horizontal incisions sutured in mattress pattern, and placed dorsally and ventrally, if more than one month prepartum. If inserted during late gestation, the suture is cut near the knot and removed at term, therefore it is vital to watch carefully for first signs of calving.

There is commonly vulvar oedema for several days. Local drainage of pus frequently occurs. A sphincter-like band of connective tissue occasionally results and may prevent future prolapse, but occasionally can cause dystocia, necessitating dorsal episiotomy (see Section 4.4, pp. 154–155).

Technique 2 **Transverse sutures**:

An inferior modification of the above method involves nylon tape which is inserted in two or three deep horizontal mattress sutures across the vulvar lips. It can produce more severe local reaction, pain and irritation, leading to continued tenesmus after analgesia wears off. There is inevitably an increased risk of sutures tearing through skin.

- insert needle with tape just lateral to the 'hairline' beside the vulvar lips
- thread suture material through or simply tie the sutures over short length of rubber or plastic tubing ('quills'), reducing risk of suture tearout

Treatment of post-parturient case

Technique 1 above is suitable. Initially in a recently calved cow, simple replacement under a long-acting (up to eight hours' duration, see Section 1.7, p. 28) epidural block is successful in most instances. Tenesmus may be further prevented by production of pneumoperitoneum (see Section 3.19 p. 138).

Technique 3   Modified Caslick's operation:

After vaginal replacement the vulvar lumen is surgically occluded over its dorsal three-quarters:

- resect vulvar mucous membrane dorsally over an area measuring about 5 cm long and 1.5 cm wide
- suture apposing surfaces with fine nylon or caprolactan (Vetafil®), supported by two deeper mattress sutures of similar non-absorbable material
- remove these sutures after two to three weeks
- incise suture line shortly before imminent parturition

Technique 4   Cervicopexy (see Figure 4.4)

Introduction

A radical method for preventing further vaginal prolapse, very effective if properly performed in the valuable non-pregnant cow. Via a left-flank laparotomy incision a suture is placed through ventral portion of cervix and prepubic tendon just lateral to midline.

Technique

- select large full-curved cutting needle and thick, non-absorbable multifilamentous suture material (polypropylene 7 metric)
- instruct assistant to apply uterine vulsellum forceps to ventral part of cervical os per vagina, pushing forceps cranially to aid identification, which is essential for correct placement, and for avoidance of urethra and bladder
- after inserting ventral cervical suture pass double length of suture material through prepubic tendon 5 cm cranial and lateral to pecten of pubis (see Figure 4.4)
- throw knots outside abdominal cavity and carry them along suture material with thumb and fingers to avoid entrapment of small intestine
- ensure minimum of four throws to each knot
- cut suture material with scissors, leaving 3 cm ends

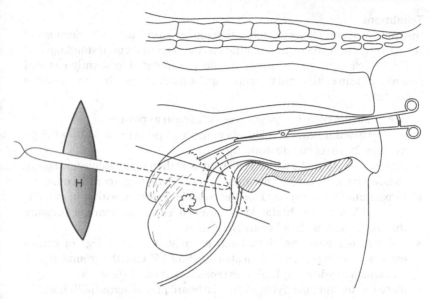

Figure 4.4 Cervicopexy through left flank laparotomy (vertical view).
A. suture through ventral part of cervix (B) which is fixed and manipulated by assistant holding long-handled uterine forceps (E) in vagina; C. point of insertion of suture through prepubic tendon; D. pubis and ventral part of pelvis (shaded); F. rectum; G. uterus; H. flank incision and suture throw; J. bladder.

This modified Winkler cervicopexy is easier and safer than the original vaginal approach.

4.3 Uterine prolapse

Introduction

Uterine prolapse occurs not infrequently (0.5% of calvings) following third stage labour, and usually involves complete inversion of the gravid cornu. Some cases follow an assisted second stage of labour. Almost unknown following caesarean section. Nearly all cases occur within fifteen hours of parturition.

Prevalent both in multiparous dairy cows in good condition (high protein intake prepartum), and in cases of malnutrition and chronic disease. Some cases predisposed by high oestrogen intake.

Aetiology unclear but uterine inversion and prolapse appear to be associated with onset of uterine atony during third stage labour. Many cows have concurrent hypocalcaemia and clinical signs of milk fever.

Treatment

Instruct farmer on phone or mobile to wrap prolapsed uterus in clean moist sheet to prevent further contamination if cow is recumbent. If standing, and sufficient help is available, uterus should be supported in slightly elevated position in clean cloths until veterinary assistance arrives. The cow should be kept quiet.

- inject calcium borogluconate s.c. or i.v. as soon as possible
- on arrival induce caudal epidural analgesia (5 ml lignocaine 2% + 0.5 ml xylazine 2%) to eliminate straining
- cleanse viscus initially with warm water and then warm saline and Epsom salts, and remove fetal membranes if already detaching spontaneously
- inspect uterus for tears and for the possible presence, within it, of a distended bladder which should be drained either by manual pressure through uterine wall, or by catheterisation
- if down, put cow into sternal recumbency with hind legs in caudal extension, to tilt perineal region at an angle of 45° with the ground, a position which considerably facilitates replacement (see Figure 4.5)
- place uterus and underlying cloth on a board placed across both hocks in recumbent cow

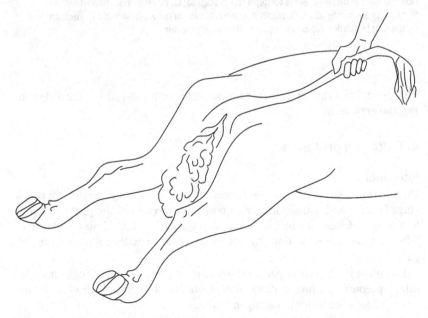

Figure 4.5 Optimal position for replacement of prolapsed uterus. Both hind legs are extended caudally. Pelvis is tilted downwards about 30° in this position. In standing cow a high epidural block may be given to facilitate manipulation.

- with the organ elevated, so that its lower edge is level with the ischium, start replacement by gentle pressure, using the palms of the obstetrically lubricated hands (KY® jelly) over the areas nearest to the vulvar lips, working in a circular manner around the mass
- practise gentle massage to avoid uterine perforation!
- after initial partial reposition, maintain reposed part by ensuring that the remaining prolapsed uterus is kept above vulvar lips
- progressively replace whole organ in this manner and ensure that it moves cranial to the cervix to its normal position
- if reposition is impossible after several minutes' manipulation locate the opening into the non-pregnant horn (usually about level with the vulva) insert the closed fist and apply firm pressure into the pelvic cavity
- check there is no residual inversion of the cornu (e.g. use empty Ca bottle as arm extension)
- if complete inversion is still impossible, fill uterine lumen with normal saline, and then siphon off through disinfected stomach tube
- after reduction inject oxytocin (50–100 iu, i.m.) to speed involution

Limited vaginal trauma can be ignored, but a large deep laceration should be sutured with catgut. Cows with extensive areas of vaginal epithelial necrosis and trauma require submucosal resection which is a haemorrhagic, slow procedure indicated only in selected cases.

Complications

Recurrence of the prolapse following return of sensation to the perineal region is uncommon. The usefulness of a Bühner pattern vulvar suture (see Section 4.2, pp. 146–147) inserted for two to three days to avoid this hazard, is controversial. Follow-up visit advisable 12–24 hours later to check vagina and cervix.

Other complications include haemorrhage, metritis, toxaemia, septicemia, paresis, and uterine rupture with bladder or intestinal eventration.

Chronic cases present problems; through and through sutures of tape or steel wire from vaginal lumen and lesser sciatic notch to skin, secured by bandage or sponge have been attempted (Minchiv method).

Prognosis for rebreeding is good and recurrence of prolapse at next parturition is inexplicably uncommon.

Amputation of the uterus (hysterectomy)

Introduction

Major surgery with rare indications, amputation is performed in cows in which the organ is so severely damaged (lacerations, necrosis, freezing, gangrene) that reposition would result in death, and in cases of prolonged prolapse in which replacement proves impossible. Amputation is sole alternative to salvage. The prognosis is guarded or poor. Major problems are haemorrhage and shock. Pre-operative whole blood or hypertonic (7.2%) saline may be advisable (see Section 1.11 p. 42). Surgery is again performed under epidural block.

Wash and prepare operative field. Two techniques are available.

Technique 1

- insert several transfixing and circumferential sutures of nylon tape just caudal to the cervix
- resect uterus about 5–10 cm caudal to this point, placing further haemostatic sutures throughout margin

Technique 2

- make dorsal incision through uterine wall to bifurcation
- identify and fan out left and right mesometrium
- ligate vessels in series, larger vessels individually, smaller vessels in groups (chromic catgut 7 metric)
- incise mesometrium 1 cm distal to sutures
- permit stumps to retract intra-abdominally
- insert mattress suture line just cranial to cervix
- amputate uterus 1 cm distal to mattress sutures
- return stump and vagina into pelvic cavity
- give systemic antibiotics for three days

Post-operative problems

Haemorrhage from uterine vessels, shock. Milking cows may remain profitable for one to two years as long as ovariectomy (see Section 4.5, p. 155) is performed at hysterectomy.

4.4 Perineal laceration

Classification

- first degree: involves mucosa of vulva/vestibule/vagina
- second degree: involves full thickness of vulva/vestibule/vagina wall, but not rectal wall or anus
- third degree: involves full depth of vulva/vestibule/vaginal walls, as well as rectovaginal tears, including anal sphincter or rectovaginal fistula

This section considers primarily third degree perineal lacerations, i.e. the most severe form.

Clinical signs

Injury is almost always a result of damage from fetal head or limbs at parturition. If possible injury can be anticipated, a veterinarian attending a dystocia case may perform dorsal episiotomy (10 o'clock or 2 o'clock position) to prevent such severe lacerations. Repair of such a surgical episiotomy wound is relatively simple (see p. 154).

Surgery is essential if breeding is to be resumed, since the severe ragged and irregular tear soon becomes oedematous and grossly contaminated by faeces. Faeces in the vagina starts a chronic inflammatory process which soon spreads to involve the cervix. At oestrus infected material may result in distortion of the shape and direction of the vaginal lumen, permitting urine pooling in cranial vagina.

Delay surgery until defect is completely epithelialised, possibly four to six weeks postpartum. Some surgeons prefer immediate surgery (not longer than four hours postpartum), but existence of inflammation and infection often leads to failure.

Technique
- keep off feed for 12–24 hours
- caudal epidural analgesia in standing animal
- cleanse surrounding area and irrigate vagina with warm disinfectant solution (povidone-iodine) and pack rectal lumen cranial to the defect with absorbent cloths
- instruct assistant to retract the lateral borders of the cloaca to expose cranially the shelf, formed by the rectal and vaginal mucosa dorsally and laterally, and supporting the underlying muscular layers
- incise transversely along caudal edge of rectovaginal shelf, and extend incision laterally to skin edge of original dorsal vulval commissure (see Figure 4.6)
- completely separate the vaginal mucosa from the edge of this shelf to a depth of about 5 cm
- suture the musculofibrous bridge, starting cranially, in a transverse plane to appose left and right surfaces (e.g. 5 or 6 metric PGA)
- start suture in the vaginal lumen and also include the four edges of vaginal mucosa
- ensure sutures are placed tight, and that their distance apart is such that it is not possible to insert a digit between them
- avoid suturing skin edges caudally (contra-indicated) since it could increase the difficulty in defaecation
- give systemic antibiotic prophylactic cover for 5 days

Problems
- inadequate mucosal undermining (a technically difficult procedure), results in an inadequate thickness of bridge
- poor placement of sutures with excessive space, permitting faecal material to pass into vagina
- sutures tearing out

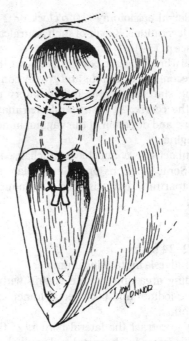

Figure 4.6 Repair of third degree perineal laceration with interrupted modified Lembert suture in dorsal layer (rectum to dorsal vagina), and continuous horizontal mattress suture in the vestibular mucosa. (From Youngquist, 1997.)

- inadvertent suture of anal skin margin causing stricture
- gross wound infection

All these problems result in partial or complete wound breakdown. Such events may necessitate a second operation. Guarded prognosis.

Dystocia is not an increased risk at any succeeding parturition.

Episiotomy

Indication
When vulva and vestibule are liable to be torn at parturition due to fetal oversize, small or immature vestibular region, or excessive friction resulting from inadequate lubrication of area. Surgical incision is preferable to a ragged, uncontrolled and bruised iatrogenic tear.

Technique
- make simple oblique incision through skin, and also vestibular mucosal layer if necessary

- avoid lengthening dorsally to anal sphincter, or cranially to damage caudal branches of vaginal artery: oblique incision should be made at 10 o'clock or 2 o'clock position
- suture incision in two layers after delivery: continuous chromic catgut in mucosa, interrupted monofilament nylon in skin
- antibiotics unnecessary

Primary healing is usual.

4.5 Ovariectomy

Indications
Alleged prolongation of lactation in mature cows as well as improvement in feed efficiency compared with non-spayed heifers. Convenient husbandry measure permitting spayed heifers and cows to run within herd with bull without risk of pregnancy. Occasionally unilateral surgery in case of ovarian pathology or persistent luteinised cyst.

Little comparative data is available regarding lactation and feed efficiency in spayed and non-spayed cattle, and much of it is contradictory.

Not widely practised in Europe, but common in parts of both South, Middle and North America, where a single surgeon, working at a restraint chute with a well-organised team, can spay 40–60 heifers an hour. Operated animals should be permanently identified.

Technique
The site for ovariectomy in a heifer (six to twelve months old) is the flank (standing) or midline caudal abdomen (recumbent). In the cow it is the vagina (colpotomy) or flank (standing).

Prior to surgery starve animal for 24 hours, no water restriction.

Flank approach
- clip left flank, wash, scrub and disinfect paralumbar fossa
- paravertebral analgesia (L1–2) or local infiltration ('T-block', 'reverse 7'), (see Section 1.8, pp. 26–27)
- practise aseptic technique: instruments and hands cleansed with quaternary ammonium disinfectant in repeated operations
- make vertical incision 10–13 cm long in left flank ventral to lumbar transverse processes 3–4
- separate muscles with scissors and incise peritoneum
- insert hand to enlarge peritoneal incision and locate ovaries
- remove ovaries with small effeminator (since ovarian pedicle is not anaesthetised by paravertebral block, swab soaked with local anaesthetic solution should be applied to pedicle for 1 minute before using effeminator). Important: do not drop either ovary into abdominal cavity!

- check that structure removed is entirely ovary
- suture abdominal wall routinely
- give systemic antibiotics for one to three days. Fly-repellant spray with residual action is indicated in warm months
- remove non-absorbable sutures in 10–14 days

Vaginal approach (cows only)

- epidural anaesthesia
- make stab incision about 5 cm long through vaginal wall at 10 o'clock or 2 o'clock position just caudal to cervix with sheathed knife (take care to avoid aorta and rectum)
- insert two fingers to locate one ovary, and draw it back into vagina
- apply local anaesthetic soaked swab to pedicle for 1 minute

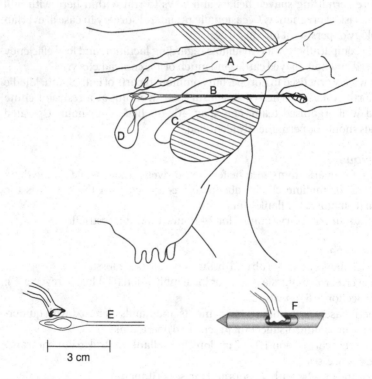

3 cm

Figure 4.7 Ovariectomy with the Willis instrument inserted through vaginal stab wound under rectal guidance. Ovary is manipulated through notch for transection of ovarian pedicle. With K-R device inner sleeve cuts ovarian pedicle while retaining ovary in lumen (see smaller illustrations).

A. sleeved arm in rectum; B. Willis instrument directed through vaginal fornix to ovary; C. bladder; D. uterine body; E. Willis instrument and close-up; F. K-R instrument.

- insert long-handled chain ecraseur or spaying shears and remove ovary (no ligation required)
- repeat on second side. No vaginal suture
- give systemic antibiotics for one to three days, possibly also analgesic

Discussion

Untoward sequelae include excessive hemorrhage from the ovarian stump especially from a granulosa cell tumour, and peritonitis.

In the USA specialized spay instruments (K-R: Jorgensen Laboratories, Loveland, CO. and Willis: Willis Veterinary Supply, Prehso, SD) (see Figure 4.7) have been developed for the colpotomy (vaginal) technique in pre-pubertal heifers (see Further Reading, Appendix 1, p. 259).

The Willis technique (see Figure 4.7) involves bilateral intra-abdominal ovariectomy via a stab incision in the vaginal fornix, using rectal palpation firstly to locate the site of proposed penetration and secondly to manipulate each ovary in turn through the sharp-edged lumen of the spay device. The ovaries are left in the abdominal cavity. With the K-R (Kimberley-Rupp) instrument, the ovary is retained in its lumen until the second ovary has been removed. Various complications have been reported (haemorrhage, bowel perforation, peritonitis).

CHAPTER 5

Teat surgery

5.1 Introduction

Intensification of dairy farming has led to earlier culling of cows with many of the teat problems discussed in this chapter ('hard milker', see Section 5.2, teat lacerations, see Section 5.5), which fail to respond to simple management such as a topical spray. In many countries treatment may be uneconomic. But in the developing world with small herds the individual cow remains a valuable resource and the owner demands maximum care and attention to teat conditions.

Significant teat injuries commonly affect the orifice, and less commonly the teat sinus wall. Teat surgery is a demanding test of the skill of the veterinarian.

Restraint and anaesthesia (see Chapter 1): xylaxine alone is very effective for minor procedures, but it is contra-indicated in advanced gestation. Beware possible recumbency! Wopa crate with one leg lifted is ideal restraint method. Local anaesthesia at the teat base, with or without sedation, and with the cow restrained in lateral recumbency, is another option.

Economic loss results from a loss in milk yield (take care with antibiotic-treated milk; possible loss of quarter if there is a necessity to dry off).

Anatomy
- teat orifice or *ostium papillare*
- streak canal or *ductus papillaris*
- Furstenberg's rosette
- teat sinus, *pars papillaris* or lactiferous sinus (teat part)
- lactiferous sinus (glandular part), milk cistern or *pars glandularis*
- teat canal: longitudinally folded stratified squamous epithelium

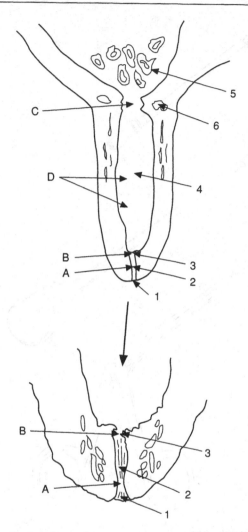

Figure 5.1 Teat anatomy and sites of stenosis.
1. teat orifice (*ostium papillare*); 2. teat or streak canal (*ductus papillaris*);
3. Furstenberg's rosette; 4. teat sinus (*pars papillaris*); 5. lactiferous sinus or milk cistern (*pars glandularis*); 6. venous plexus.
Sites of teat obstruction: A. tight streak canal; B. obstruction at Furstenberg's rosette; C. milk cistern obstruction (proximal stenosis); D. teat sinus obstruction.

- teat sinus: superficial columnar, deeper cuboidal epithelium; below mucosa is layer of embryonal-type cells capable of rapid proliferation
- muscularis, subcutis and skin

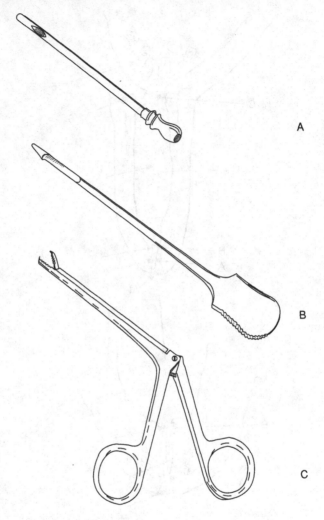

Figure 5.2 Teat instruments.
A. milk catheter for passive milk drainage; B. Hug lancette for opening or dilating the streak canal; C. Teat alligator forceps for the removal of 'milk stones', either free or attached to teat mucosa, through the streak canal.

5.2 Stenosis of teat orifice, streak canal or Furstenberg's rosette

Aetiology
Common problem. Partial obstruction ('hard milker') due to local trauma, possibly secondary to milking machine malfunction (e.g. excessive vacuum

pressure) or microtraumatic wounds sometimes permitting the development of *Fusobacterium necrophorum* infection ('blackspot').

Signs
Quarter milks out slowly, or 'valve' is evident, and vicious cycle may develop as remaining quarters tend to be overmilked, resulting in bruising and eversion of teat orifice and development of mastitis. Some cases are inoperable.

Treatment
Controversial, and there are no controlled studies on efficacy of method.

Non-infected case (i.e. no mastitis) and **non-inflammatory** teat orifice lesion:

- in mild cases consider simple insertion of self-retaining canula (Naylor® teat dilator) for five days, without surgery, alternatively insert Larsen® teat tube
- alternatively tense orifice between finger and thumb, cleanse with iodophor solution
- insert Maclean's® teat knife, D-D (Dyakjaer-Danish), Hug® (see Figure 5.2), or Lichty® (blunt point) knife once and withdraw rapidly
- check adequacy of milk flow and if poor, re-insert knife at 90° to original incision
- if flow is still poor, insert teat bistoury and thereby cut out plug of teat canal
- insert self-retaining teat canula for five days; initially rotate canula gently every few hours to avoid development of excessive granulation tissue
- as alternative to teat canula, tie cow up and remove milk from the quarter several times every two to three hours for the first two days
- give intramammary antibiotics prophylactically for five days (N.B. milk withdrawal)
- instruct stockman to roll end of teat regularly before applying machine

Infected case (i.e. with mastitis and/or severe inflammatory reaction):

- treat with intramammary antibiotics and local application of antibiotic cream before attempting surgery

Treatment of choice: remove obstructing tissue in Furstenberg's rosette or streak canal during thelotomy, or, if available, with theloresectoscope (see Figure 5.3). Return to normal machine milking in 75% of cases

5.3 Teat lumen granuloma

Introduction
Also known as 'pea' or 'spider', this lesion is a discrete proliferation of granulation tissue covered by mucosa and caused by trauma, which initially causes a submucosal haematoma projecting into teat cistern.

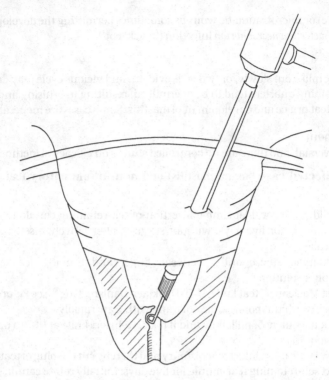

Figure 5.3 Theloresectoscopy. Scope is introduced into teat sinus through lateral teat wall incision. Stenotic tissue around Furstenberg's rosette is removed with the cautery sling.

Signs
Often asymptomatic but can eventually cause interference with free passage of milk, is rarely pedunculated, but painless.

Treatment
Complete removal is often difficult, and recurrence rate is high!

- attempted blind removal via mosquito or long alligator forceps, teat bistoury, or fixation and traction by Hudson's spiral, often causes further trauma
- logical approach in case producing clinical signs is open surgery (thelotomy) in lateral recumbency following ring block: vertical incision in teat wall opposite mass, and resection by scalpel. Suture in three layers, mucosa with fine continuous absorbable material, then wall, finally skin. Teat wound heals well if careful, sterile technique is adopted
- milk daily using sterile teat cannula (passive milk drainage)

- return to machine milking of quarter on day eleven
- drying off quarter is often best option

5.4 Teat base membrane obstruction

Congenital form occurs in some heifers; acquired form is in cows, usually at start of new lactation, aetiology unknown, possibly inflammation of basal annular membrane.

- teat lance or Hug's knife (see Figure 5.2b) is inserted in attempt to break down the annular membrane

Prognosis is very poor and treatment usually hopeless.

5.5 Traumatic lacerations of teat

Introduction
Factors affecting outcome and prognosis include:

- involvement of streak canal
- direction of wound: longitudinal wounds heal better than transverse
- integrity of blood supply
- presence of infection
- amount of skin loss

Treatment
Superficial wounds: basic surgical principles apply and all wounds must be regarded as contaminated.

- thorough gentle cleansing with non-irritant dilute antiseptic, e.g. povidone-iodine or chlorhexidine
- leave superficial wounds unsutured, but dress with bland antiseptic cream, e.g. chlorhexidine gluconate (Savlon™, Schering-Plough) or proprietary mixture of propylene glycol and organic acids (Dermisol® cream, Pfizer) after débridement of traumatised and avascular tissue with fine sharp scissors and rat-tooth forceps
- some cases benefit from taped dry dressing (e.g. Elastoplast® Smith & Nephew) to appose wound edges

Deeper wounds involving muscularis and skin:

- suture after cleansing, irrigation and débridement
- insert continuous sture into muscle layer with monofilament absorbable metric 2
- insert skin sutures, simple interrupted of metric 2 polypropylene
- cover wound over with Opsite® (Smith & Nephew) after spraying with Leukopor® ('New Skin' spray)

Local antibiotics: apply only to skin suture line, never to wound surfaces, where they delay healing. Use penicillin + streptomycin (Streptopen® Schering-Plough) or oxytetracycline hydrochloride (Terramycin® Pfizer) in powder, cream or aerosol preparations.

Use of routine intramammary antibiotic is controversial.

Passive milk drainage for ten days before resuming machine milking

Problems include excessive suture tension, which causes puckering and skin necrosis, and poor healing resulting from inadequate débridement or cleansing of lesion.

Teat laceration involving teat sinus

Introduction

Fistulae are usually acquired. Treat recent (< 12 hours) fistulae by immediate surgery (primary wound healing). Repair older wounds by tertiary wound healing, (e.g. 10–14 days post-trauma or during dry period). Prognosis is guarded.

Work in good operating facilities, with adequate light, cleanliness and efficient analgesia. Ensure stockman understands post-operative care.

Surgical technique

- cleanse with non-irritating antiseptic
- trim off devitalised skin, muscularis and mucosa
- appose or invert mucosal edges, but suture submucosa and muscularis with interrupted sutures of 3 metric PDS on swaged-on needle. Do *not* suture mucosa!
- suture skin with simple non-absorbable (e.g. polyamide 2 metric) interrupted mattress sutures to produce precise apposition of edges
- use of protective bandage and self-retaining impregnated cannula for several days is controversial, and lacks comparative studies (e.g. 'Opsite'®)
- perform passive milk drainage every one to two days (depending on quarter yield), and insert intramammary preparation every second day
- healing takes about ten days, when sutures are removed. Cases of wound breakdown should be re-operated at the earliest possible moment in the dry period.

Causes of breakdown

- severe post-operative oedema
- poor suture technique
- excessive suture tension
- necrosis of wound edges
- infection

Local non-surgical treatment with organic acid, butter of antimony and, most recently acrylics and electrocautery, usually fails to close a teat fistula.

5.6 Imperforate teat

Aetiology is congenital in heifers, or acquired as a result of trauma in adult cattle.

Assess whether milk is present in teat sinus; surgery is only indicated in positive case. Proceed as for teat stenosis (see Section 5.2, pp. 160–161).

5.7 Incompetent teat sphincter

Aetiology is invariably traumatic in case of a single teat, which constantly or intermittently leaks milk.

Treatment
- difficult and indicated only in chronic case (> 3 weeks) as fibrosis of granulation tissue repair may correct condition spontaneously
- inject minute volume of irritant drug (e.g. sterile Lugol's iodine) with tuberculin syringe around teat orifice (e.g. 4 × 0.1 ml) to stimulate discrete circumferential fibrosis

Technique is hazardous and results unpredictable.

5.8 Teat amputation

Supernumerary teats

Introduction
Congenital and inherited condition. The teats tend to be small, are commonly caudal, but sometimes are attached to the normal teat. Remove when one to nine months old, and never within one month of parturition (oedema, wound breakdown, infection, mastitis). Up to three months old, removal may be performed by unqualified but trained person, but under anaesthesia. UK law requires that surgery in calves over three months old be performed by veterinary surgeon under anaesthesia. Swiss law requires all ruminant surgical procedures to be performed by veterinarian under anaesthesia. Many countries have no legislation to cover this, and many other specific procedures.

Technique
- carefully identify supernumerary teats
- small calves: resect with scissors
- in older calf crush at base with small Burdizzo® (Emasculatome) and resect with knife along inner edge of blades
- line of section should be cranial to caudal, not transverse, so that subsequent scar merges into natural folds of udder skin
- suture only if wound edges separate

Amputation due to disease

Indicated in severe purulent or gangrenous mastitis of one quarter to permit drainage, also following irreversible teat damage.

Technique
- analgesia of teat base and application of good restraint
- place Burdizzo® at junction of middle and distal thirds of teat, amputate with scalpel distal to jaws
- retain teat lumen by continuous sutures in wall (skin to mucosa) using interlocking mattress suture to maintain drainage

Haemorrhage is usually slight.
Quarter will eventually dry off as a result of secondary infection and mastitis.

Amputation due to injury

Introduction
Teat amputation may also be indicated in cows with severe teat damage where reconstructive surgery and return to normal function cannot be expected, e.g. loss of distal portion of teat, or long, oblique or transverse tears into teat canal. Amputation and closure of teat sinus is only successful in the absence of infection.

Technique
- amputation site is 1–2 cm distal to udder-teat junction
- transect teat by scalpel, resecting the mucous membrane 1 cm below the cut surface
- invert mucosa by continuous suture in submucosa (see Figure 5.4)
- insert horizontal mattress sutures to close musculature and appose skin edges with simple sutures or metal clips (Michel)
- infuse antibiotics into the quarter before final sutures are placed.

In gangrenous mastitis, following teat amputation at the junction with udder, a cruciate incision is made into udder skin to permit optimal drainage and exposure to atmosphere to inhibit anaerobes. Irrigation with dilute H_2O_2 is useful.

5.9 Discussion

Meticulous care to details of technique is vital in surgical repair of severe traumatic teat lesions. A multiplicity of suture patterns illustrates the unsatisfactory results obtained in certain hands, but this is more likely to be a result of deficiencies and breakdowns in basic surgical principles, than to any defect in the suture configuration itself.

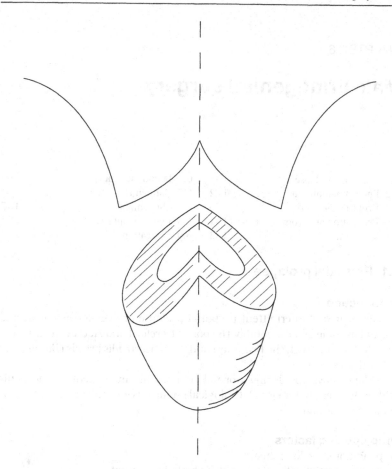

Figure 5.4   Teat amputation with primary closure: cut surfaces for closed teat amputation.

Dedicated aftercare by stockman and veterinarian is of major importance for success.

Aftercare of teat surgery includes passive milk drainage for ten days, frequency depending on yield, intramammary antimicrobials every second day, a clean environment for wound and cow, and removal of sutures about day eleven.

Apart from wound breakdown and local infection, mastitis remains the major hazard, and up to 40% of teat-traumatised cows are culled for mastitis within, or at the end of, that particular lactation. Amputation of accessory digits (prophylactic) preventing teat injury is discussed in Chapter 7 (see Section 7.12 p. 225).

CHAPTER 6

Male urinogenital surgery

6.1 Preputial prolapse

Introduction
A mild degree of intermittent preputial prolapse or eversion is considered normal in some breeds, notably the polled Hereford and Aberdeen Angus in the UK, together with the Brahman and Santa Gertrudis breeds (*Bos indicus*) in North America.

Prolapse develops during normal non-erectile movement of the penis within the preputial cavity. Pathological prolapse is more likely in individuals exposed to trauma.

Predisposing factors
- pendulous and long sheath
- large preputial orifice with limited ability to contract
- poor development of the preputial and retractor penis muscles in some polled breeds (see above)

Preputial trauma
Pathological prolapse is more likely in individuals at range or pasture exposed to trauma, which may involve irritation from foreign bodies such as vegetation, dust or earth, and which are secondary to penile injury.

Common site of injury is the mucosa adjacent to skin-prepuce junction. Frostbite can cause major problems in certain areas in the winter. All cases of preputial prolapse should have complete physical examination of the external genitalia.

Sequence of events following injury is:

- severe localised oedema and hyperaemic congestion
- extensive fibrosis with secondary infected fissures and cracks
- areas of granulation tissue develop in the cracks with secondary infection

- as a result, penile erection may be abnormal, with only the glans tip passing through this damaged region

Another common site of preputial trauma leading to prolapse, is the reflection of parietal prepuce on to the body of the penis. It may be sustained during natural or artificial service.

Conservative treatment
Recent injury to prolapsed mucosa may be treated conservatively:

- carefully cleanse the area with non-irritant dilute antiseptic solution (povidone-iodine)
- soak damaged prepuce in swabs containing 25% magnesium sulphate solution to reduce oedema
- apply emollient dressing (e.g. zinc and castor oil ointment) and replace prolapse
- place purse-string suture in preputial orifice or if the prepuce is too oedematous to be reduced a polyvinyl tube (2.5 cm diameter and 15 cm long) is placed in the preputial lumen and wrapped firmly with elastic tape
- tape is applied directly to the tube and the skin on the sheath beginning at the preputial orifice and extending toward the abdominal wall
- placement of tube decreases oedema and permits escape of the urine
- systemic antibiotics and anti-inflammatory drugs for five days, as well as local antibiotic irrigation
- dress any prolapsed preputial mucosa with lanolin-based ointment and keep covered to prevent further trauma

Radical surgery: circumcision
Cases with secondary diffuse fibrosis and excoriation require surgery in lateral recumbency, under sedation and ring block local analgesic infiltration, or general anaesthesia (see Section 1.9, p. 36). A rubber band tourniquet may be applied proximally to decrease haemorrhage.

Two circumcision techniques are used commonly in bulls:

- resection and anastomosis, also known as posthioplasty or reefing
- surgical amputation, resulting in the loss of equal amounts of external and internal lining of the prolapsed portion of prepuce, performed using suture or ring technique

Four potential post-operative complications must be recognised before surgery is attempted:

(a) prepuce can be made too short for breeding: this depends on the breed but, as a general criterion, the usable prepuce must be twice as long as the free portion of the penis
(b) surgeon should remove only the diseased prepuce

(c)   circumferential scar (cicatrix) contraction can result in phimosis

(d)   post-operative haemorrhage can lead to dehiscence and infection

1 Resection and anastomosis technique

- close clip and shave the hair from the distal portion of the sheath and preputial orifice
- if penile extension is possible, place towel forceps in the apical ligament or alternatively have an assistant hold the penis
- scrub and prepare the prepuce and penis
- place two marking sutures proximal and distal to the area of prepuce to be removed to ensure that the prepuce is aligned anatomically when sutured
- examine the prepuce and make circular incision through the epithelium of the prepuce proximal to the area to be resected
- deepen this incision until normal tissue is observed
- make a second circular incision distal to the area to be removed. In *Bos indicus* bulls, it usually is necessary to resect at least 15 cm of prepuce to prevent recurrence of the prolapse. In *Bos taurus* bulls, as much prepuce as possible should be salvaged
- connect these two circular incisions then with two longitudinal incisions
- remove the pathological portion of prepuce by sharp dissection. It is important to control any haemorrhage, because even small haematomas could induce wound dehiscence
- ligate any large veins or arteries
- lavage the surgical site copiously with saline solution
- extend and retract the penis until the two incisions are in apposition thus ensuring that the penis is freely movable. The two marking sutures also should be aligned
- if the elastic tissue has been incised appose it using interrupted sutures
- close the epithelium with a simple interrupted pattern
- suture a 4 cm diameter Penrose drain to the free portion of the penis with three or four interrupted sutures of catgut; place sutures superficially to avoid the urethra. The Penrose drain will direct urine away from the incision line during the healing period
- insert a gas-sterilised 15 cm section of 2.5 cm polyvinyl tube into the prepuce with the Penrose drain through it
- attach the tube to the sheath with elastic adhesive tape and completely enclose the incision. The adhesive tape can be sutured to the skin to prevent premature dislodgement of the tube. Presence of tube decreases oedema formation and aids in the prevention of stenosis
- inject antibiotics for a minimum of five days after surgery
- remove the bandage and tube five to seven days after surgery
- replace the tube and bandage if penile prolapse occurs. Vigorous attempts to extend the penis and inspect the surgical site should not be made until three weeks after surgery

- do not remove the preputial sutures because such attempts may damage the surgical wound
- keep the bull from breeding for at least 60 days when, if possible, the animal should be evaluated to make sure the penis is extendable without restriction of the prepuce. Oedema of the prepuce usually persists for ten days after surgery. NSAIDs and diuretic agents can be used if oedema is excessive

2 Technique of surgical amputation

- often performed when penile extension is not possible because of phimosis or adhesions
- clip and prepare aseptically the area of the end of the sheath
- attach two Backhaus towel clamps to the distal end of the prepuce
- place a finger inside the prepuce
- insert horizontal mattress sutures full thickness around the prepuce immediately proximal to the area of amputation: these mattress sutures should overlap one another through both layers of the prepuce to control bleeding; tie tightly
- amputate prepuce through an oblique line to create an oval orifice
- appose the edges of the prepuce with a simple interrupted pattern
- suture a Penrose drain to the penis and insert a tube into the prepuce and attach with elastic tape

The post-operative management is similar to the first technique. A v-shaped incision at the ventral aspect of the preputial orifice can be made to reduce the risk of phimosis.

A modification of the amputation technique has been described in which as much as possible of the unaffected inner aspect of the prolapsed prepuce is left and only the external aspect affected by the inflammatory process is removed. This is especially crucial in *Bos taurus* breeds.

3 Preputial amputation with ring

Preputial amputation using the ring technique involves the insertion of a plastic ring into the preputial cavity. This technique can be advantageous to the practitioner with limited facilities. The ring and sutures act as a tourniquet, and the prepuce distal to the ring will necrose in about 14 days. The ring is made from a tube 5 cm long and 4 cm in diameter with 1 mm holes drilled through the wall spaced 5 mm apart at the midpoint. The ends of the tube should be smooth, and the tube should be sterilised.

- place the bull in lateral recumbency
- place the plastic ring into the preputial cavity so that the holes are located at the desired point of amputation
- put a ligating suture pattern around the prepuce through the holes in the ring using non-absorbable suture material and tie every suture tightly

- amputate the prepuce 5 mm distal to the suture line. Minimal haemorrhage is observed if all sutures have been tightened sufficiently
- extend the penis through the plastic ring and suture a Penrose drain to it
- return the penis, prepuce and ring to the preputial cavity and place a purse-string suture at the preputial orifice to prevent prolapse
- after two weeks remove purse-string suture and pull the ring out; necrotic tissue and sutures are often still attached to the ring. The ring may slough spontaneously during this period
- sexual rest is recommended for 60 days after treatment

Intra-preputial adhesions

Introduction
Intra-preputial adhesions present problems in exposure, evaluation and management. Exposure may be very difficult and accompanied by tearing of the adjacent preputial mucosa.

Degree of mechanical hindrance caused by the adhesions may be hard to evaluate since, though some adhesions will be palpable, others will not. Adhesions are frequently obliquely longitudinal rather than circumferential.

Surgery
- remove mucosa overlying the adhesions between circumferential incisions
- resect all fibrotic adhesions down to the *tunica albuginea* (TA)
- carefully appose mucosal edges, as in the first technique (see p. 170)

Bull should be rested for two to three weeks, depending on degree of post-operative oedema, and can then be teased with increasing frequency (initially every three days, later daily) to prevent recurrence of fibrosis and adhesions.

Prognosis is guarded or poor depending on area resected.

6.2 Penile haematoma

Introduction
Condition is more accurately termed rupture of the *corpus cavernosum penis* (CCP) with a rent in the *tunica albuginea* (see Figure 6.1), through which blood explodes into the surrounding tissues.

Vigorous, over-enthusiastic thrusting at intromission, or possibly spontaneously during masturbation. Penis may undergo severe downward bending leading to tear in *tunica albuginea* (TA). Alleged higher incidence in horned English breeds (e.g. Hereford).

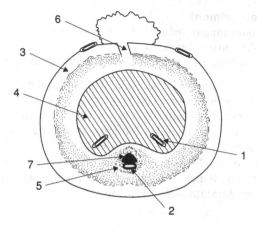

Figure 6.1 Cross-section of penis just distal to distal flexure (sigmoid) to show haematoma site.

1. deep veins of penis; 2. artery of penis; 3. *tunica albuginea*; 4. *corpus cavernosum penis*; 5. *corpus cavernosum urethrae*; 6. usual site of penile haematoma, with blood from *corpus cavernosum penis* escaping through dorsal tear in *tunica albuginea*; 7. urethra.

Pathology

Site is immediately prescrotal and usually dorsal, close to insertion of the retractor penis muscles near the distal flexure of the sigmoid. Rupture of CCP causes immediate haematoma which may grow over a few days to a variable extent as a result of slow leakage. Lesion may be strictly localised or relatively diffuse. Secondary preputial oedema and preputial prolapse may occur, rarely with some penile protrusion. Compression of lymphatic and venous drainage may cause secondary preputial prolapse.

The natural course of penile haematoma is a gradual reduction of the swelling, as oedema disappears and the haematoma is slowly organised into fibrous tissue. A significant proportion of cases of penile haematoma however develop a serious complication – an abscess at the site (often *Arcanobacterium pyogenes*) and a fibrous adhesion – and the prognosis is then grave.

Abscessation usually leads to a fluctuating swelling to one side of penis, separate from penile body. Avoid exploratory paracentesis, which can result in iatrogenic infection of a sterile haematoma.

Differential diagnosis

- preputial prolapse of primary origin
- penile injury of other aetiology
- urethral rupture due to occlusion by calculus

Conservative treatment

Small haematoma rapidly reduces in size, is often hard to detect ten days later, and requires no treatment.

A larger haematoma may resolve following medical treatment:

- remove bull from herd and ensure sexual rest for 60 days
- give systemic antibiotics for seven days
- apply hot packs, cold water sprays, or possibly ultrasound; all these methods lack controlled studies but have allegedly reduced the healing period, but also increase the degree of fibrosis
- after 30 days manually extend penis and check sensation of free portion. Lack of sensation indicates bilateral nerve damage and bull will neither breed nor ejaculate into artificial vagina

Surgery

Due to the possibility of infection entering the haematoma and causing abscessation, surgery is often advisable for all cases, except smaller haematomata (< 20 cm) that rapidly resolve.

- place bull on systemic antibiotics as soon as possible following injury
- note that long-term systemic chemotherapy (oxytetracyclines, sulphon-amides) has been alleged adversely to affect fertility
- operate with aseptic technique under GA (preferable to sedation and local infiltration analgesia)
- starve for 48 hours, and no water for 24 hours
- place bull in lateral recumbency
- aseptic preparation of affected area which should be draped throughout surgery
- incise laterally through skin of sheath into lateral aspect of CCP over haematoma
- carefully evacuate haematoma of all clotted blood by blunt dissection with fingers and gentle curettage (Volkmann's double curette, or spoon curette)
- exteriorise penis proximal to haematoma to inspect distal part of sigmoid flexure, where source of haemorrhage may sometimes be identified
- remove any superficial blood clots from region and bluntly dissect through elastic tissue to identify rent
- if possible, suture tear in TA after débridement of edges with simple interrupted sutures of 5 metric PGA
- irrigate haematoma cavity with three mega crystalline penicillin G dissolved in 20 ml normal saline, and appose wall of haematoma cavity
- similarly close subcutaneous tissues in simple continuous pattern with PGA after assistant has grasped and extended penis to maximum degree
- close skin incision with interrupted non-absorbable simple or mattress sutures
- maintain bull on systemic antibiotics for five days after surgery

- avoid insertion of drains in attempt to reduce post-operative accumulation of serum

Tease bull after three weeks to discourage development of scar tissue and adhesions of subcutaneous tissues to the penile body. The bull may be returned to service after 60 days. The prognosis is guarded, but about 75% return to natural breeding with surgery.

Complications
Temporary seroma formation, abscessation, adhesions to sheath, nerve damage, (with desensitisation of glans penis) vascular shunt formation, recurrence of injury, and preputial injury from secondary prolapse.

6.3 Urolithiasis

Introduction
Calculus is a clinical problem in entire but more frequently in castrated male cattle. Triple phosphate calculi are found in cattle on concentrate feed; and silica calculi (e.g. North America) in cattle on high silica pasture grass or hay.

Urolithiasis is not a problem in female cattle due to their relatively larger urethral diameter, though severe cystitis occasionally results from a bladder packed with calculi.

Clinical signs
- lodgement at proximal or distal part of sigmoid flexure, distal 30 cm of penis, or over ischial arch
- initial straining with partial or complete urinary obstruction
- clinical cases are dull and feed intake is reduced, and after the initial 24 hours of obstruction straining ceases
- pressure necrosis of urethral mucosa and eventual urethral rupture with seepage of urine into subcutaneous tissues of the ventral body wall and possibly scrotum is possible
- rupture of bladder, often in dorsal cranial part of fundus but occasionally near bladder neck, and gradual accumulation of intra-abdominal urine is another possibility ('water belly')
- subcutaneous accumulation of urine, which should be treated by incisional drainage, eventually results in skin slough as blood supply is impaired, leaving moist area of granulating tissue (30–40 cm diameter) in which the penis may be identified and from which urine drips (mild uraemia)
- following complete urinary obstruction, and bladder rupture, cattle remain comparatively bright; blood urea increases after three days at a rate of about 10 mmol/litre/day, with death from uraemia and associated metabolic problems after seven to ten days.

Treatment

Emergency surgery may be undertaken in uraemic cattle, with the aim of economic salvage several weeks later when there is no metabolic abnormality and the surgical wounds have healed. In rare cases an attempt is made to preserve the breeding capacity of a valuable bull by urethrotomy, but surgery is seldom successful for several reasons:

● precise location of calculus may be difficult to establish
● several calculi may be present at different sites, necessitating multiple incisions
● suture of the urethral wall is awkward, as attempts at simple apposition, with minimal stenosis, frequently result in urinary seepage through the incision

Resuturing is unlikely to be more successful:

● fibrosis and chronic stenosis are common sequelae, eventually leading to recurrence of blockage by several smaller calculi

Intra-urethral insertion of a polypropylene catheter to a site proximal to the incision and protruding through the glans, has been attempted. In this technique urethral sutures pass through the muscularis and outer serosal layers only. Catheter is removed five to seven days later.

Urethral obstruction caused by one or more calculi lodged in the sigmoid region should be relieved by a midline incision in the caudal dorsal aspect of the scrotum, i.e. the ventral perineal region. The sigmoid, which is relatively mobile, may be exteriorised for palpation and surgery.

Ruptured bladder

Diagnosis is based on:

● rectal palpation – bladder cannot be appreciated
● abdominal ballottement for fluid thrill
● abdominal paracentesis (midline, most ventral site, 2.1–1.65 metric needle)

Treatment

As a first step abdominal urine is drained slowly (approximately 2 litres/5 minutes) via ventral abdominal cannula attached externally to wide-bore tubing and screw clips (to adjust flow rate). This drainage may start before preparation for laparotomy. Rapid reduction of intra-abdominal pressure imposes unnecessary cardiovascular stress as abdominal venous bed dilates.

If general condition permits, left flank laparotomy is done standing, otherwise in right lateral recumbency.

● paravertebral analgesia L1–3 (see Section 1.8, pp. 22–24)
● make vertical left flank incision 20–30 cm long in caudal paralumbar fossa

- grasp bladder with right hand and explore surface with left hand – rupture is frequently found dorsal and cranial. Rupture more caudally, involving bladder neck and trigone area, is extremely difficult to repair surgically
- evert bladder and examine mucosa especially of neck, to assess severity of cystitis and to remove any calculi
- calculi detected in peritoneal cavity are harmless
- confirm patency of distal urinary tract (i.e. urethra) by flushing saline via catheter inserted through bladder neck, around ischial arch; in case of urethral obstruction further surgery is indicated (see above and below)
- place continuous inversion suture (Lembert or Cushing pattern) in bladder wall using 7 metric chromic catgut
- close body wall routinely (see Section 3.3, Closure of flanklaparotomy Incision p. 86), disregarding residual abdominal urine
- ensure good flank wound apposition, removing blood and urine from flank musculature

Alternative technique for salvaging steer or bull with dorsal and cranial bladder rupture relies on spontaneous healing of this wound (see Figure 6.2).

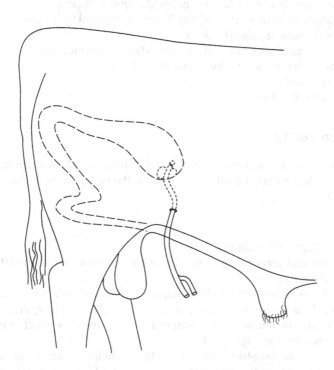

Figure 6.2 Implantation of Foley catheter into urinary bladder for temporary drainage in urolithiasis in male cattle. Catheter exits the abdominal cavity to the right of the prepuce.

- perform right flank laparotomy
- pass mushroom-headed rubber (Foley) catheter from outside through ventral body wall, following stab incision through skin to grasp catheter tip with forceps within abdomen
- make stab incision in vertex of bladder
- insert catheter through stab incision and inflate balloon with 15 ml NaCl to keep catheter in place
- ensure that catheter is slightly curved within the abdominal cavity to avoid possible displacement during movement such as standing up, and to allow for some growth
- anchor catheter to skin
- remove catheter only if normal urine later passes through the urethra, otherwise leave in place until salvage some weeks later
- give systemic antibiotics to all cases following ruptured bladder – poor risk cases benefit from i.v. fluids (10–20 litres)

Complications of bladder surgery
- death from circulatory failure and metabolic disturbance
- bladder wall breakdown resulting from poor surgical technique
- severe chronic haemorrhagic cystitis
- blood-borne or ascending infections leading to pyelonephritis
- urethral stenosis and renewed bladder rupture
- atony of bladder
- diffuse peritonitis

Urethrostomy

Urethrostomy, i.e. a permanent urethral fistula, is indicated in complete urethral obstruction at level of, or distal to, the ischial arch. It is a salvage operation.

Technique
- caudal epidural analgesia
- routine skin preparation from anus to scrotal neck and about 10 cm to each side of midline
- midline skin incision from dorsal aspect of ischium distally for 15–20 cm
- blunt dissection around distal part of root and proximal body of penis; the crura are surrounded by the ischiocavernosus muscles which meet in a midline *raphé* (see Figure 6.3)
- incise penis longitudinally, precisely in midline (otherwise urethra will be bypassed), separating bulbo-urethral and ischiocavernosus muscles

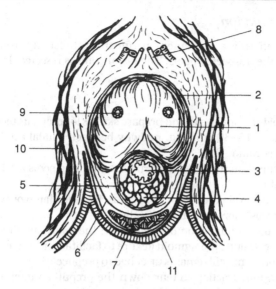

Figure 6.3 Horizontal section through perineal region of steer to indicate structures in perineal urethro(s)tomy.
1. *corpus cavernosum*; 2. *tunica albuginea*; 3. urethra; 4. *corpus spongiosum*; 5. *tunica albuginea* of *corpus spongiosum*; 6. perineal fascia; 7. retractor penis muscle; 8. dorsal artery, vein and nerve of penis; 9. deep artery of penis; 10. medial muscles of thigh; 11. skin.

- enter urethral lumen 0.5–1.5 cm deep to muscular surface, after incising the surrounding *corpus cavernosum urethrae*. Inevitably some haemorrhage occurs from the related venous bed. Cattle with a grossly distended bladder and a patent pelvic urethra void urine through the incision at this point
- extend incision distally 2–6 cm, depending on patient size
- suture urethral mucosa and minimal depth of fibrous tissue component of erectile tissue to skin with 5 metric PGA attached to swaged-on needle
- place initial sutures dorsally and ventrally, then suture laterally
- place indwelling catheter (flexible polypropylene with large lumen, 5–10 mm external diameter) into bladder and suture to skin through encircling tape
- flush bladder via catheter daily with dilute povidone-iodine solution (0.1%) and remove catheter after three days

Incision site is very dorsal and avoids problem of catheter tip impinging on distal orifices of the ducts of the bulbo-urethral glands, which lie dorsolaterally in urethral mucosa. Size of urethrostomy should prevent significant stenosis resulting from scar tissue contraction.

Penile amputation

Involves creation of a permanent perineal urethrostomy from the proximal part of the transected penis. The distal penis is resected. It is a salvage operation.

Technique
- caudal epidural analgesia, and prepare skin as for previous technique
- skin incision 15–30 cm long, midway between caudal aspect of scrotal neck and ischium
- isolate penis from surrounding structures, pulling penis forcibly through skin incision
- identify the fine pink retractor penis muscles, and clamp proximally with artery forceps before sectioning distally
- continue upward direction of traction on the penis and dissect bluntly, with fingers around the sigmoid flexure to facilitate easy exteriorisation of this portion; penis still remains attached to prepuce
- either continue traction to tear down the preputial attachment to skin at the preputial orifice, or incise the preputial tissues with scalpel and scissors just caudal to skin-preputial junction; leave preputial orifice unsutured
- transect completely exteriorised penis after ligation at a point estimated to permit about 10 cm protrusion of the penile stump through the skin wound
- ligate dorsal artery and vein of penis, situated cranially in stump, with 7 metric chromic catgut
- incise urethra proximally from cut end for 3 cm to produce a flared spatulate end to hinder stenosis
- place PGA sutures through each side from external fibrous coat into urethral mucosa for haemostasis
- suture penis into skin edges so that stump protrudes about 5 cm at angle of 30° to horizontal
- appose remaining subcutaneous tissues and skin by monofilament nylon sutures
- give systemic antibiotics for five days. Clean the penile stump twice daily for three days.

Further haemorrhage occasionally requires additional ligation.

Discussion
Ventral abdominal subcutaneous accumulation of urine resulting from urethral rupture can be drained via multiple stab incisions.

Complications include slow continuing haemorrhage and development of stenosis. In some cases a misdirected flow of urine causes soiling of the skin of the hind legs.

6.4 Prevention of intromission

Introduction

Various methods have been developed to prevent intromission (insertion of the penis into the vulva and vagina of the female) in cattle. One method, penile translocation, is outlined as a possible surgical technique (see below). Several techniques may be unlawful in some countries, and unethical in others.

Other surgical techniques to prevent intromission include:

- penectomy: penis transected and exposed in perineum
- phallectomy: penis shortened by removing distal extremity, but organ remains in preputial cavity
- penopexy: penis transfixed to abdominal wall ventrally or to ventral perineum via sigmoid flexure
- preputial obstruction: prosthetic device fixed in orifice, preventing extrusion of penis, or insertion of purse-string suture at the preputial orifice with creation of a preputial fistula ventrally for the urine to escape

Reference to these specialised techniques may be found in Appendix 1 pp. 259–260.

Penile-prepuce translocation

Introduction

Translocation (or transposition) of the penis is used in production of teaser bulls. Operation is combined with vasectomy or epididymectomy to render the animal sterile. Translocation avoids the hazards of possible spread of venereal disease by preventing intromission. It is claimed that libido is maintained. Surgery should be done well before the breeding season in animals ideally 250–300 kg. Operation creates a new preputial opening into which the penis and prepuce are sutured. Surgery is performed in dorsal recumbency under GA or deep sedation with local analgesia.

This form of surgery on normal cattle has been forbidden in the UK under the Welfare of Livestock (Prohibited Operation Regulations) Act 1982.

Technique

- the aim being to redirect the penis 30° laterally, usually to the right, mark the proposed site on the skin in the standing bull. The place is usually at the level of the fold of the flank (see Figure 6.4)
- following anaesthesia and turning bull into dorsal recumbency, clip and disinfect the new site and the preputial region for an aseptic procedure
- irrigate preputial cavity with a dilute (1%) povidone-iodine solution and close orifice with purse-string suture (infection risk!)

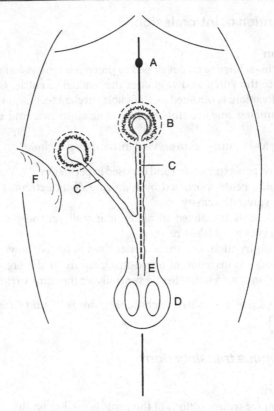

Figure 6.4 Penile and preputial translocation in young bull ('teaser bull'), ventral view, lines of skin incisions around prepuce, penis and new body wall site are shown as interrupted lines (––––––––).
A. umbilicus; B. skin-prepuce junction in midline; C. penis; D. scrotum; E. level of sigmoid flexure; F. fold of right flank.

- remove 8 cm diameter circle of skin from the new site and cover temporarily with a moist sterile swab
- make corresponding incision around preputial orifice, having marked (e.g. with temporary suture) cranial midline point, and continue dissection close to midline caudally
- elevate the preputial coat from the body wall and ligate the extensive vascular supply
- stop dissection at distal part of the sigmoid flexure; this tunnel may be advantageously started with long-handled straight scissors
- cover prepuce with sterile glove before pushing it into subcutis

- carefully avoiding any torsion on the penis or prepuce and noting cranial midline point previously marked, place preputial skin in new site and move penis into appropriate position along abdominal wall (see Figure 6.4)
- insert a series of interrupted chromic catgut sutures in the subcutaneous tissues
- suture skin with simple interrupted sutures of monofilament nylon
- close midline skin defect similarly, but include several deeper sutures into *linea alba* and rectus sheath to avoid creation of potential dead space
- five-day course of systemic antibiotics
- perform epididymectomy (see Section 6.6, pp. 185–186) or vasectomy (see below).

Three weeks after surgery several ejaculates (approximately three) should be evaluated to ensure that bull is safe for use as 'teaser'.

6.5 Vasectomy

Introduction
A portion of ductus deferens is removed from the spermatic cord on the cranial aspect of the scrotal neck (see Figure 6.5). This technique is practised

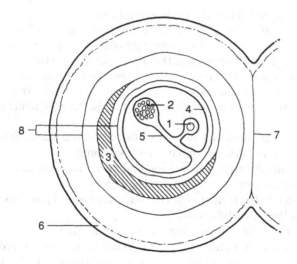

Figure 6.5 Diagrammatic cross-section of scrotal neck (left side) showing relationship of vas deferens, vascular supply including pampiniform plexus, and cremaster muscle, to vaginal tunics.
1. vas deferens enclosed in internal *tunica vaginalis*; 2. vasculature (pampiniform plexus and spermatic artery) in internal *tunica vaginalis*; 3. cremaster muscle; 4. external *tunica vaginalis*; 5. internal *tunica vaginalis*; 6. skin; 7. scrotal septum (*tunica dartos*); 8. internal and external spermatic fascia.

to produce a teaser bull. Intromission is unaffected, giving the risk of transmission of venereal disease.

Surgery may be attempted in the standing animal (if it is not combined with penile translocation procedure), but is easier if bull is recumbent with the hind legs extended caudally, or in lateral recumbency with the upper hind leg held well forward, (as for equine castration). The risks of GA in bulls should be borne in mind.

Anaesthesia
Standing method: xylazine sedation (low dose range, i.e. 0.1–0.15 mg/ kg i.m.) followed by local infiltration with 10 ml 2% lignocaine injected subcutaneously around proposed incision site, carefully avoiding possible injection into pampiniform plexus.

Recumbent method: xylazine sedation (high dose range, i.e. 0.2 mg/kg i.m.) supplemented by local infiltration.

Surgical technique
• clip hair from entire upper half of the scrotum and scrotal neck
• scrub and thoroughly prepare scrotum and adjacent skin for aseptic surgery
• apply povidone-iodine twice to the scrotal skin
• make vertical incision 5 cm long on caudolateral (if standing) or craniomedial (cast) aspect of lower part of scrotal neck over tensed cord structures. In standing position the skin must be rotated through 90°
• grasp spermatic cord between thumb and first two fingers and gently rotate to identify ductus deferens as very firm thick string or wire-like structure about 4 mm diameter (it is the hardest structure in the cord)
• carefully make small nick in vaginal tunic over the ductus deferens and place hook beneath it, or grasp in Allis tissue forceps
• bring ductus through skin incision and clamp across with two pairs of artery forceps about 5 cm apart (see Figure 6.6)
• resect intervening section of ductus with scissors and place silk ligatures (3 metric) below each forceps
• release forceps; ligature avoids possible recanalisation
• retain ductus for identification (e.g. examine for semen) and possible histopathology, as potentially useful evidence in eventual litigation
• close skin incision with interrupted horizontal mattress sutures of monofilament nylon
• repeat surgery through second incision on other side
• give systemic antibiotics for five days
• check bull for absence of semen by teasing once weekly for three weeks
• remove skin sutures after 10–14 days

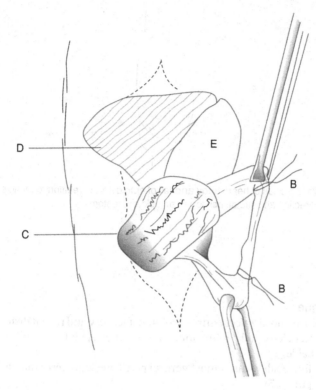

Figure 6.6 Vasectomy in recumbent bull. Vertical incision in lower scrotal neck and cord structures elevated by scissors (see also Figure 6.5).
A. cord-like ductus (vas) deferens in internal *tunica vaginalis*, held by Allis forceps; B. non-absorbable sutures ligating ductus before resection of 5 cm; C. adjacent pampiniform plexus; D. cremaster muscle; E. fold of *external tunica* vaginalis incised to expose A. and C.

6.6 Epididymectomy

Introduction
The tail of the epididymis is resected. Resected tissue must be checked for semen, since, inadvertently, only fat and connective tissue may be removed. Surgery can be done in standing bull under xylazine sedation and local infiltration. Strict asepsis is essential.

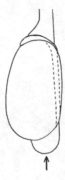

Figure 6.7 Location of head, body and tail of epididymis in relation to testicle. Arrow indicates direction and site of incision in an epididymectomy.

Technique

- clip, wash and disinfect entire scrotal surface; dry and repeat disinfection
- push testicle distally with one hand so that epididymal tail is readily identifiable
- incise into epididymis at most ventral point, avoiding testicular substance (see Figure 6.7)
- grasp large portion of tail with Allis forceps and place large artery forceps transversely proximal to this tissue, which is then resected
- place firm suture of PGA (7 metric) proximal to the artery forceps which is then removed
- insert two to three horizontal mattress sutures to appose skin edges
- give systemic antibiotics for five days
- remove sutures in 10–14 days
- tease bull weekly for three weeks when no live sperm should be seen; bull is then suitable for work

Discussion

Again portions of epididymis removed at surgery should be retained as a precautionary measure should litigation materialise, based on a claim that a bull has remained fertile. Recanalisation is impossible following the above techniques, in which the lumen of the ductus and epididymis are occluded by encircling ligatures.

Sclerosing agents have also been injected into the testicle and epididymis of bulls to produce fibrosis and to abolish spermatogenesis and sperm transport. They are less reliable than surgical methods.

6.7 Congenital penile abnormalities

Corkscrew penis or spiral penis

Introduction
This congenital defect, involving the apical ligament, occurs in bulls older than one year. Many affected bulls are known to have served successfully, and have sired progeny. Any breed can be affected, but polled breeds such as polled Hereford have a higher incidence. Inheritance is questionable.

Signs
- seen just before or immediately following extrusion of the penis from the sheath
- in severe cases the penile tip is caught in distal part of preputial cavity and may only be extruded naturally with some difficulty
- extruded penis spirals to left or right through 30° angle, viewed from the right side, and 180–270° when viewed (theoretically) from the rear
- glans penis tends to hit right perineal region of cow, about 20–30 cm from the vulva

Spiralling action may be variable in degree; in intermittent cases bulls may maintain a low level of fertility in the field. In normal bulls, occurrence of deviation and complete spiralling after intromission increases the contact area between the penis and vagina, and may therefore increase tactile stimuli and so promote ejaculation. In affected bulls the deviation or complete spiralling occurs prior to intromission and prevents coitus. Anatomical explanation involves slipping of the dorsal apical ligament across to the left and ventrally. The penile integument in affected bulls is then fully stretched over the penis and produces spiralling early in the process of copulation.

As long as the inheritance remains questionable, surgery should only be undertaken after consideration of the ethical position, and then reserved for valuable bulls required for natural service.

Surgical techniques
Two techniques are given, one using penile *tunica albuginea* (TA) the other with *fascia lata* from the thigh region.

Technique 1 Penile *tunica albuginea* (see Figure 6.8):
- GA, lateral or dorsal recumbency
- extend penis, avoiding accidental spiral rotation, and apply rubber tourniquet at base
- grasp glans with forceps or tie with bandage, and maintain penis in full extension

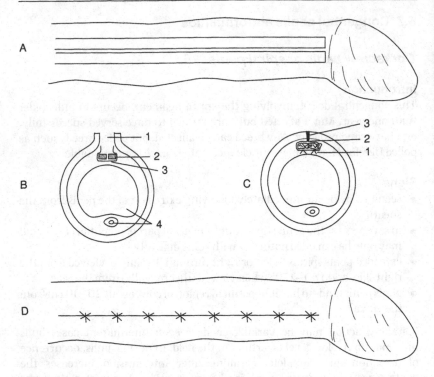

Figure 6.8 Surgical correction of spiral deviation of penis ('corkscrew penis').
A. dorsal surface of penis with epithelium incised and two strips (each 10 cm × 2 mm) of apical ligament freed from *tunica albuginea* (TA) except proximally
B. cross-section of penis showing (from dorsal): 1. incision through penile epithelium; 2. two sections of dorsal ligament (shaded); 3. incision in TA; 4. *corpus cavernosum penis* and urethra ventrally
C. enlarged cross-section showing position of sutures fixing strips of apical ligament to TA; 1. sutures from strips to TA; 2. suture closing TA over strips; 3. closure of penile epithelium
D. interrupted sutures closing penile epithelium.

- make dorsal midline incision through penile mucosa from just cranial to reflection of prepuce forwards to just caudal to glans
- expose underlying dorsal ligament of penis
- incise longitudinally through middle of ligament into TA
- incise 3 mm laterally to left and right, parallel to previous incisions
- incise transversely and distally across distal end of previous three incisions so creating two strips (2 mm wide) of ligament and TA
- resect about 1 cm of strip length and re-attach strips to distal end of dorsal ligament with alternate sutures of 6 metric chromic catgut and 3 metric stainless steel (respectively to provoke a tissue reaction and for strength)

- strip is tacked on to underlying fibrous coat with interrupted sutures every 6–7 mm, ensuring firm contact and deep insertion into TA
- close penile epithelium with 4 metric chromic catgut interrupted sutures
- irrigate wound with aqueous solution of penicillin G and release tourniquet
- give antibiotics systemically for five days
- close preputial orifice temporarily by encircling muslin bandage for some hours until bull has recovered from anaesthesia and can retain penis in preputial cavity
- irrigate preputial cavity daily with oleaginous antibiotic preparation from day four to day ten
- sexual rest for eight weeks, then tease bull to ascertain new position of erect penis

Technique 2   Fascia lata graft:

- general anaesthesia
- fix the bull in right lateral recumbency

First collect the *fascia lata* graft as follows:

- clip and prepare a liberal area from the proximal tibia to the *tuber coxae* for surgery
- make an incision beginning 8 cm dorsolateral to the patella and continued for 20 cm toward the *tuber coxae*, continue the incision to the *fascia lata* of the *vastus lateralis* muscle
- collect a 3 cm wide and 20 cm long rectangular strip of the deep *fascia lata*. Remove connective tissue from the strip, and keep graft in saline; (homogenic *fascia lata* preserved in 70% ethyl alcohol also has been used successfully to reduce surgical time and avoid a second incision on the patient)
- close fascial layers in a simple continuous pattern and appose skin with non-absorbable suture material in routine fashion
- extend the penis manually, and prepare the penis and prepuce for aseptic surgery
- make a 20 cm skin incision on the dorsum of the penis starting about 2.5 cm proximal to the tip
- deepen the incision to the white fibrous apical ligament
- reflect the apical ligament laterally in both directions, exposing the TA
- do not incise the two veins on the right ventral aspect between the ligament and the TA
- place the *fascia lata* graft between the apical ligament and the TA on the dorsum of the penis
- insert four interrupted sutures of 2 metric polyglactin 910 through the *fascia lata* and into the TA under the ligament, near its origin
- then place interrupted sutures along the lateral margin of the graft at 2.5 cm intervals to stretch the implant

- trim the implant to fit the distal end of the penis and suture under tension in an interrupted pattern
- return the apical ligament over the implant and suture it with a simple interrupted pattern of the same material; the thickest portion of the ligament should be on the dorsum of the penis
- close the last layer with 3 metric polyglactin 910
- insert a tube into the preputial cavity and secure to the sheath with elastic tape to maintain the penis in a retracted position
- give systemic antibiotic agents for three to five days
- maintain sexual rest for 60 days

In some cases (resulting from over- or under-correction) a second operation is required. The prognosis remains guarded.

Persistent frenulum

Introduction
Congenital anomaly. Persistence of embryonic ectodermal lamella connects penis to the penile part of prepuce, which usually splits after the calf is two months old, and in which completion is hormone-dependent, but may be delayed until eight months. Excessive thickness of ventral bridge (= frenulum), perhaps containing blood vessels, may be an aetiological factor.

Signs
Band of fibrous tissue runs from close to penile tip to near junction of penile part of prepuce and sheath, causing marked ventral deviation of erect penis. This prevents intromission.

In the USA it is most common in Aberdeen Angus and Shorthorn bulls, but has low incidence.

Treatment
- ligate blood vessels in frenulum and section fibrous structure with scissors

Good prognosis. Condition possibly inherited, therefore ethics of surgery are dubious.

Other congenital anomalies of bovine penis

These include:

- congenitally short penis (infantile)
- congenitally short retractor penis muscle
- congenitally tight penile adnexa

All three conditions have a low incidence. The main sign is that penis fails to reach vulva despite normal erection. No surgical correction possible.

6.8 Penile neoplasia

Penile tumours occur in two forms, papillomatosis or fibropapilloma, and malignant squamous cell carcinoma.

Papillomatosis

Occurs in young bulls, reared in groups. Aetiologically a host-specific Papovavirus, (BPV_1).

Signs
- haemorrhage from penis, often on turning out to cows or at breeding examination
- located on free portion of penis; generally multiple and sessile, but chronic cases may have pedunculated mass
- phimosis or paraphimosis is possible

Treatment
- slow spontaneous regression can occur
- autogenous wart vaccine usually unsuccessful
- surgical removal (knife or Burdizzo®), electrocautery or cryosurgery
- unless simple procedure, patient should be in lateral recumbency to facilitate precision
- sedation with xylazine
- analgesia by local infiltration of dorsal nerves of penis (see Section 1.8, p. 31) or subcutaneous ring block
- care required not to open urethra (potential fistula formation)
- ligate or cauterise significant bleeding vessels
- close epithelial defect with 0 metric chromic catgut (not essential)

The prognosis is good.

Malignant squamous cell carcinoma

Malignant SCC is a rare condition in adult bulls, usually rapidly invasive and involving multiple ulcerating and proliferating masses. Histopathology for confirmation? Surgery usually impossible and prognosis correspondingly poor.

6.9 Castration

Introduction
Need for castration has been increasingly questioned on scientific, economic and humanitarian grounds. Two forms of castration are available: bloodless and open surgical (scalpel).

Bloodless methods

Rubber ring method

This method should not be used, nevertheless this technique is becoming more common in some areas. The technique has been ethically condemned in the UK and is illegal without anaesthetic in some countries (e.g. Germany, Switzerland). Legally in the UK a rubber ring, without anaesthetic, is only permitted in the first week of life.

Application of tight-fitting rubber ring to scrotal neck in calves appears to cause considerable post-operative discomfort and marked setback to growth. Some sepsis is not uncommon at site following skin necrosis. Careless application can fail to position both testes below rubber ring, resulting in induced (iatrogenic) inguinal cryptorchidism. It also carries a risk of tetanus, probably as the duration of pressure necrosis is much greater than in other bloodless methods.

In the USA rubber band tubing has even been used, especially in feedlots, for the castration of large bulls. The ring is applied with the EZE® Bloodless Castrator (Wadsworth Mfg., Dublin, MT). As in the calfhood method a vascular necrosis of the scrotum and testes results. The authors have no experience of this technique which is alleged to result in 'minimal stress'.

Analgesia

In the UK, legislation (Animal Anaesthetics Act 1964) makes it obligatory that castration of calves over two months old be performed under anaesthesia or analgesia.

In Switzerland castration without anaesthesia is forbidden.

- 10 ml syringe and 2% lignocaine (with adrenaline)
- testicle is grasped between thumb and first two fingers and drawn to ventral part of scrotal sac
- needle is introduced in horizontal or vertical position, upwards into substance of testicle, and 3 ml solution is injected
- testicle is released and 2 ml is deposited in subcutaneous position during withdrawal
- procedure is repeated on the second side

An alternative technique involves subcutaneous infiltration at scrotal neck, injection of a further 3–5 ml into each cord, because one author (AS) believes that intratesticular injection is painful, minimally effective and should therefore be avoided. Maximum dose rate of lignocaine is 4 mg/kg bodyweight.

Burdizzo® method

The Burdizzo® instrument is 30 or 40 cm long, and has cord stops. It is used on calves one to twelve weeks old, depending on breed and development.

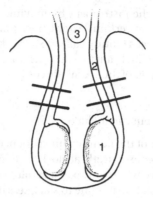

Figure 6.9 Diagram of vertical section through scrotum, showing correct position for application of Burdizzo® (bloodless) emasculator. Cord is pushed laterally to produce minimal skin trauma. Area of undamaged skin is left in midline and maintains blood supply to ventral part of scrotal skin. The instrument is applied remote from penis. 1. testicle; 2. spermatic cord; 3. penis.

- surgeon stands beside the calf, keeping the hindquarters against a suitable pen wall with the head placed and tied or held in a corner by assistant
- surgeon controls the correct application of the Burdizzo® (see Figure 6.5): the instrument is applied laterally onto the scrotal neck by assistant behind calf
- cord is held laterally in scrotal neck by first finger and thumb of surgeon
- the second hand controls position of the jaws; instruct assistant initially to close the jaws slowly until they are about 8–10 mm apart and are about to clamp skin and cord firmly
- with cord precisely located between the jaws, order rapid closure
- maintain closed for 5–10 seconds, during which operator checks that cord is correctly crushed
- characteristic crushing sound accompanies the closure. Cord-stops on the emasculator blades help to prevent displacement of the cord during closure
- separate jaws 1 cm, slide them 1 cm distally, and close a second time on the same side. In contrast to the first crushing, there is minimal pain reaction
- repeat the procedure on the second side
- ensure that the crushed lines in the skin are offset (see Figure 6.9) and do not form a continuous band around the scrotal neck which could otherwise lead to skin necrosis with infection. Do not crush the median (scrotal) raphé.

Another Burdizzo® model has a knee grip. In this technique the assistant restrains the hindquarters, while the surgeon holds the cord in position with one hand while closing the instrument by moving one handle against the knee-fixed second handle. A certain dexterity is required.

The effect after four weeks (young calf) or six weeks (older calf) is atrophy of the testicular tissue, which forms a fibrous knob or knot-like structure approximately the diameter of the spermatic cord.

Complications
Problems are infrequent but can include:

- inadvertent crushing of the penis by inexperienced lay operator, as jaws are applied too high, causes urethral blockage and rupture with s.c. urine seepage. Salvage procedure is only possible solution
- gross bruising of scrotal tissues due to slackness of jaws, therefore equipment should be regularly overhauled and the instrument should be stored in the open position. Burdizzo® should be capable of cutting piece of string inserted between two pieces of cigarette carton card when functioning normally
- necrosis of scrotal skin (see above)
- oedema of caudal abdominal wall and scrotum due to slack jaws
- unilateral absence of testicular atrophy, as cord was inadvertently completely or partially missed

Surgical (scalpel) method
This technique involves removal of the testicles and haemostasis of the spermatic cord vessels by:

- traction on spermatic cord
- torsion and traction on spermatic cord
- crushing using an emasculator
- crushing and ligation of spermatic cord

Technique
- perform surgery in standing position with stockman restraining head and hindquarters and holding tail laterally
- induce local analgesia, as described above
- wash and cleanse scrotal skin with dilute (0.5%) povidone-iodine solution, and preferably wear disposable gloves
- stand or crouch behind calf to make vertical incision through caudal scrotal skin into testicular substance, holding testicle tensed and pulled distally, and continue incision along distal, i.e. ventral border of scrotum (ensuring subsequent drainage)
- scrotal incision should be slightly shorter than testicular length.

Initial scrotal incision may be made with Newberry® knife (Newberry® castrating knife, Jorgensen Labs, Loveland, CO. USA), a 24.5 cm long instrument with steel-bladed clamp) which is placed transversely across

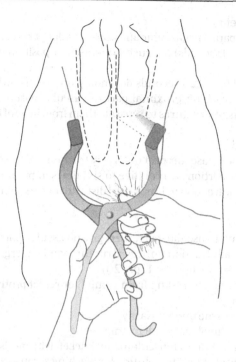

Figure 6.10 Newberry castration technique. View from rear, showing testes pushed upwards, scrotum pulled down by hand, and Newberry knife being applied across scrotum for transverse incision, before being pulled quickly downwards. Dotted lines represent the position of the *tunica vaginalis*, through which the testes are then extracted.

the base of the scrotum, closed, and immediately pulled ventrally to open both scrotal sacs without removal of any scrotal tissue (see Figure 6.10). Both testicles may then removed with the emasculator.

- testicle prolapses through skin wound, is grasped, and vascular and non-vascular portions of the cord are identified (vascular: cranial including pampiniform plexus and vas deferens)
- insert first finger through *tunica vaginalis* proximal to the epididymis, and between vascular and non-vascular parts.

Technique now varies depending on method of haemostasis:

- small calf (one week to two months): emasculator, torsion, traction are possibilities in descending order of preference
- large calf (two to six months): emasculator, torsion. Traction is contra-indicated as excessively painful
- small bull: emasculator, possibly with ligation

All other methods carry a risk of severe haemorrhage.

Emasculator method
- apply after separating vascular and non-vascular parts of cord
- brief period (10 seconds) to crush non-vascular position just proximal to epididymis
- longer period (20–120 seconds depending on size of cord and the age of the animal), crushing proximal part of vascular portion of cord, using traction on distal structures to separate them from jaws of instrument

Torsion method
- break down non-vascular part of cord by traction
- twist vascular portion several (five to six) times in proximal part of cord, then use gentle traction to break cord distal to torsion point

Traction method
- break down non-vascular part, then grasp vascular portion proximally, increasing steady traction until cord ruptures and undergoes considerable elastic recoil (see Section 3.11, p. 120)
- repose any tissue protruding from wound, or resect protruding length of *ductus deferens*
- do not handle tissue unnecessarily
- do not become involved in calf restraint
- maintain scalpel and emasculator in bucket with antiseptic and have second bucket of antiseptic solution for washing scrotum
- local medication is unnecessary

Technique for small bull
Emasculator and ligation; strict aseptic precautions and antiseptic preparation of skin are essential. Use sterile emasculator and suture material.

- incise as above, caudally, into substance of scrotum, continuing incision distally
- apply emasculator to non-vascular part of cord, then to vascular portion, close tightly and remove testis
- leave instrument in place for minimum of 1 minute
- place circumferential ligature around cord 1 cm proximal to blade, as extra security against haemorrhage
- place artery forceps on edge of cord proximal to ligature but not across cord, remove emasculator, and check for haemorrhage
- release artery forceps

Ensure clean bedding. Some exercise is advisable for one week.

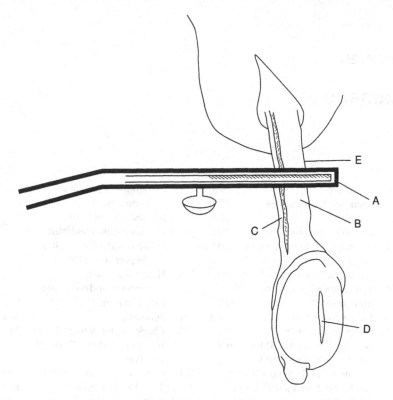

Figure 6.11 Emasculator castration (diagrammatic). Scrotum has been incised distally into testis which has then been expressed from scrotum. Parietal *tunica vaginalis* has been sectioned by scalpel and has retracted into scrotum.
A. Emasculator placed across cord structures with cutting edge of blade distal and crushing edge proximal ('nut' to 'nut'); B. *pampiniform plexus* and spermatic artery; C. *ductus deferens*; D. testicular incision; E. site for application of artery forceps to retain stump for a few seconds' inspection if warranted.

Complications

- infection – gross contamination at surgery, (rubber gloves!) dirty bedding
- severe swelling – infection, oedema, poor drainage due to small incision
- haemorrhage
- preputial oedema – invariably from extension of scrotal swelling
- tetanus is rare (prophylaxis in at-risk calves)

CHAPTER 7

Lameness

Systemic infections such as Foot-and-Mouth disease (FMD) and clostridial diseases, metabolic conditions such as ketosis and hypomagnesaemia, as well as nutritional diseases (e.g. hypovitaminosis E), are not considered in this book although they may lead to signs of lameness.

7.1 Incidence

Veterinary practice figures (UK) indicate an average annual incidence of 4–6% lameness in dairy cows. If treatment carried out by the farmer is included, however, the true incidence increases to 25–30%. The incidence may range from 3–100% on individual farms. Any farm with an incidence over 15% should be considered to have a lameness problem which requires systematic investigation (see Section 7.16). In the intensive agricultural enterprises common in western Europe and North America:

- 95% of lame cattle are dairy breeds
- 80% of cases involve the digits
- 80% of digital lameness is located in the hindlimbs
- 50% of digital lameness involves the horny tissue and 50% the skin, mostly digital dermatitis
- 70% of the horny lesions involve the outer claw

In the UK today the three major digital lameness problems with rather similar incidence rates, are digital dermatitis, sole ulcer, and white line disease. The latter two may sometimes be related to a previous incident of laminitis.

Essential equipment for investigation of bovine lameness problems includes:

- facilities for good restraint and ready elevation of hind- or forelimbs ideally purpose-built for foot work e.g. Wopa crush/chute or a rotating model
- good lighting, hosepipe, water, bucket, brush, and ropes
- left- and right-handed hoof knives
- double action hoof cutters
- hoof rasp
- hoof testers
- straight grooved probe
- grinder for large-scale (i.e. herd) trimming with electrical cut-out in case of short-circuiting

7.2 Economic importance

Only infertility and mastitis cause greater economic losses than lameness in most intensive dairy units in the UK, western Europe (Netherlands, Denmark, Belgium, Germany) and North America. The 2004 estimate of UK losses due to cattle lameness is well over £100 million (US $180 million). In developing countries infectious diseases and malnutrition are of more economic importance.

Economic losses

The direct cost of each lameness case is about £150 ($270), but if such factors as prolonged calving interval, replacement costs and culling losses are included, the figure rises to approach £300 ($540) for each lame cow in a national herd of about three million dairy cows (UK). Losses are similar in USA.

Losses result from:

- reduced milk yield
- weight loss

- disposals, deaths, replacement cost
- infertility, prolonged calving interval
- veterinary expenses, drugs
- additional stockman's time

A major loss is reduced **milk yield**, including discarded antibiotic-treated milk during therapy period. This accounts for about a quarter of all losses due to lameness. Lameness is primarily in the early lactation period (one to three months postpartum) and in the immediate prepartum week. This time of maximum incidence results in greater economic losses than lameness in mid or late lactation. Several studies have shown that higher yield cows tend to have an increased risk of lameness, also that a reduction in yield actually precedes lameness onset. No satisfactory explanation has been found for these two (UK) facts. Cash loss due to a lameness successfully cured within 24 hours of onset may represent 1% of lactation yield. If treatment is delayed, loss may be 20% or more of lactation yield.

Weight loss may be 10% or, in cows eventually culled due to continuing deterioration and poor yield, may reach 25%.

Disposals as 'lame cow culls' in the UK are about 2–4% annually, but such lame cows are often also affected with mastitis and/or metritis leading to infertility. The replacement cost for culls is considerable.

Infertility attributable to lameness results from:

- failure of oestrus detection (cow often recumbent, unwilling or unable to mount neighbouring cows) or delayed return to oestrus
- anoestrus
- poor body condition postpartum (negative energy balance)
- concurrent low grade metritis

These losses are subtle, and often not fully appreciated by the dairy farmer, but are the greatest source of cash loss (see Figure 7.1).

Veterinary expenses and drugs form a small proportion of total costs. The additional labour costs, often ignored, are high since treatment usually involves two or three people, and each case requires several minutes' attention, often on a daily basis (see Figure 7.1).

Hoof traits
Variations in hoof traits relate to survival rates, reproductive performance, and increased yield from first to subsequent lactations (see Section 7.14 pp. 231–232).

7.3 Terminology

Terms have been introduced to give an acceptable terminology to forms of lameness common to various countries, where a variety of words have been

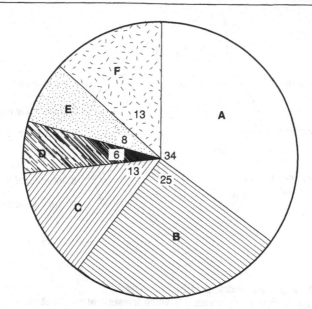

Figure 7.1 Economic losses in dairy cattle due to lameness: A. infertility; B. reduced milk yield and sales; C. deaths, disposals and replacements; D. weight loss; E. veterinary expenses, drugs; F. cost of extra labour.

in use. The Latin terms are listed beside the English language equivalent (and illustrated in Figure 7.2).

Interdigital skin:

- digital dermatitis – *dermatitis digitalis*
- interdigital necrobacillosis – *phlegmona interdigitalis*
- interdigital skin hyperplasia – *hyperplasia interdigitalis*
- interdigital dermatitis – *dermatitis interdigitalis*
- verrucose dermatitis – *dermatitis verrucosa*

Horny tissues:

- solear ulceration – *pododermatitis circumscripta septica*
- punctured sole – *pododermatitis septica (traumatica)*
- white line separation – *pododermatitis septica diffusa* (disputed)
- laminitis – *pododermatitis aseptica diffusa*
- longitudinal (vertical) or transverse (horizontal) sandcrack – *fissura ungulae longitudinalis et transversalis*
- heel erosion – *erosio ungulae*

For further details see Further Reading, pp. 259–260.

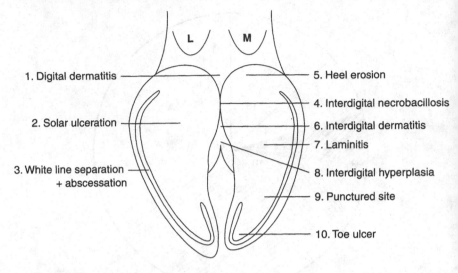

1. Digital dermatitis
2. Solar ulceration
3. White line separation + abscessation
5. Heel erosion
4. Interdigital necrobacillosis
6. Interdigital dermatitis
7. Laminitis
8. Interdigital hyperplasia
9. Punctured site
10. Toe ulcer

Figure 7.2 Important conditions of the bovine digit.
1. digital dermatitis; 2. sole ulceration; 3. white line separation and abscessation;
4. interdigital necrobacillosis; 5. heel erosion; 6. interdigital dermatitis; 7. laminitis/sole
haemorrhage; 8. interdigital hyperplasia; 9. punctured sole; 10. toe ulcer.

Claw zones

The bearing surface of the claw has been divided into six zones to aid recording (see Figure 7.3). Thus white line separation and abscessation tends to be in zones one or two, sole ulcer in zone four, and laminitic changes predominantly in zones four and five.

Lameness scoring (LS)

Many numerical scales (e.g. 0–3, 1–6, 1–10) have been devised and utilised in recording the severity of lameness in an individual cow. The simplest appears adequate, viz. 0 = not lame; 1 = slightly lame; 2 = moderately lame, and 3 = severely lame/often recumbent (e.g. LS2).

7.4 Interdigital necrobacillosis

Introduction

Synonyms: *phlegmona interdigitalis*, 'foul-in-the-foot', 'clit ill', 'foot rot', interdigital pododermatitis. A peracute form, colloquially 'superfoul' has been encountered in some countries recently.

Definition: acute inflammation of subcutaneous tissues of interdigital space and adjacent coronary band, spreading to dermis and epidermis.

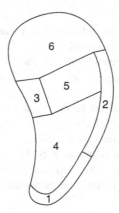

Figure 7.3 Zones of the sole.
1. white zone at toe; 2. abaxial white zone; 3. axial groove zone; 4. apex of sole;
5. junction of sole and bulb (heel); 6. bulb (heel).

Signs

- mild to severe lameness (LS 1–3) of sudden onset, all ages
- interdigital swelling, later involving coronet and pastern
- toes spread apart due to interdigital swelling, initially with unbroken skin for first 24 hours of lameness
- sometimes more proximal spread, and a secondary interdigital necrosis very common
- little pus but characteristic foul smell and pain with split in interdigital skin

Aetiology: interdigital microtrauma and infection with *Fusobacterium necrophorum*, *Bacteroides melaninogenicus* and other organisms.

Pathology: cellulitis and liquefactive necrosis of interdigital skin, with fissure formation and later, if untreated, development of granulation tissue, eventually resulting in interdigital granuloma. Advanced cases can develop digital septic arthritis and other deeper complications. The disease course is much more rapid in 'superfoul' where cows may have to be culled 48–72 hours after disease onset, due to the extent of destructive changes.

Differential diagnosis: interdigital foreign body, acute laminitis, solear penetration by foreign body, severe interdigital dermatitis, interdigital changes from BVD/MD, FMD, distal interphalangeal septic arthritis, distal phalangeal fracture.

Treatment
- ceftiofur, ampicillin, LA oxytetracycline, penicillin, sulphonamides (e.g. trimethoprim-sulpha) systemically
- clean affected necrotic area with disinfectant and apply a topical oxytetracycline or copper sulphate, or BIPP paste (bismuth subnitrate, iodoform and petrolatum)
- do not bandage, but put on to dry floor or straw bedding, preferably isolated to avoid spread of infection
- daily cleansing with disinfectant if feasible
- 'superfoul': early cases respond well to 6 g oxytetracycline, more advanced cases to tylosin, careful local débridement under analgesia and local antibiotic dressing. Isolation is important.

Prophylaxis
- check and improve drainage in areas where interdigital trauma can arise (e.g. gateways, tracks, stubble)
- improve dry conditions underfoot (straw yard) and increase frequency of scraper removal of slurry from passageways
- footbaths of zinc sulphate (5–10%) copper sulphate (5%) or formalin (4%) (see Section 7.15, pp. 234–235)
- antibacterial feed additive: sulphabromomethazine in feedlot outbreak, or ethylenediamine dihydroiodide for prophylaxis, though results have been conflicting (North America)
- spread quicklime in muddy tracks or around water troughs

Discussion
Frequent form of digital lameness (e.g. 15% of total), but of relatively lesser economic importance since the 1980s. Outbreaks of interdigital necrobacillosis require methodical investigation of aetiology to develop appropriate prophylactic measures. Emphasis on major areas for digital trauma (from yard to parlour to farm tracks) and for potential contamination. Review claw trimming needs.

7.5 Interdigital skin hyperplasia

Introduction
Synonyms: *hyperplasia interdigitalis*, corn, interdigital granuloma, interdigital vegetative dermatitis, fibroma, 'wart'.

Definition: proliferative reaction of interdigital skin and/or subcutaneous tissues to form a firm mass.

Incidence: usually sporadic, common in certain beef breeds (e.g. Hereford) and in bulls at AI centres. Occasionally follows severe interdigital disease in dairy cows, then is unilateral. May start in yearling bulls, but most clinical cases (with lameness) are in adults of four to six years.

Predisposition: inherited in some breeds (e.g. Hereford, Holstein Friesian). Severe interdigital dermatitis or sole ulcer often precedes involvement of single limb. Frequently associated with poor conformation e.g. splayed toes with wide interdigital space.

Signs
- slight or no lameness (LS 0–1) depending on size and mechanical interference in simple case
- large lesions develop superficial digital traumatic ulceration, and contact interdigital axial skin may undergo pressure necrosis
- both forms readily become secondarily infected with *Fusobacterium necrophorum*
- more or less symmetrical in hindlimbs of beef breeds, especially in bulls, possibly with bilateral forelimb involvement, which suggests inherited basis
- single abaxial hindlimb involvement suggests secondary response to recognised previous insult involving interdigital swelling and sometimes sole ulcer

Pathology: skin hyperplasia with secondary ulceration. Variable degree of hyperkeratosis (misnamed papillomatosis).

Differential diagnosis: interdigital foreign body, interdigital necrobacillosis, digital dermatitis.

Treatment
- none if small and asymptomatic
- local caustic (e.g. silver nitrate, copper sulphate) if small and causing lameness
- most clinical cases require resection by knife surgery electrocautery or cryosurgery: ideally in Wopa crush under IVRA (intravenous regional analgesia), bandage (e.g. Vetrap®) after applying sulphadimidine powder. Remove bandage after one week.

Discussion
Acquired cases develop suddenly in middle of interdigital space; while congenital cases, manifest as slight swelling in yearling and steadily enlarging with adulthood, start as fold in the axial skin of the abaxial digit. Theoretically, breeding policy should be altered to reduce the inheritance risk of such cases of multilimb hyperplasia. Inheritance may be related to skin thickness, an alleged slackness of the interdigital cruciate ligaments and the amount and distribution of body fat.

7.6 Solear (solar) ulceration

Introduction
Synonyms: *pododermatitis circumscripta*, sole ulcer, Rusterholz ulcer.

Definition: circumscribed limited reaction of the pododerm (deep sensitive tissues) often characterised by an erosive defect typically at the sole-heel junction of the lateral hind claw.

Incidence: high (up to 40% of digital lameness cases) and widespread in dairy breeds, from calved heifers to mature cows in good body condition.

Aetiology: disputed, possibly excessive weight-bearing by lateral claw following horn overgrowth. Associated almost invariably with abnormal claw (poor trimming), and frequently with laminitis. Primary and secondary causes are difficult to distinguish.

Predisposition: inherited factors such as stance, which may also be acquired, and deviations from normal hoof shape (e.g. severe overgrowth), loose housing with small (narrow, short) cubicles, giving tendency for cows to stand with hind feet in passageway, overgrown digits, acidotic rations.

Signs
- moderate degree of lameness (hesitant, wary gait, slightly arched back, LS 1) typically up to three months postpartum, masking the frequently bilateral nature of the lesions, i.e. lateral claw of both hind legs, one more painful than the other
- severe lameness (LS 2–3) when granulation tissue protrudes and in presence of deeper purulent infection (osteomyelitis, septic arthritis)
- under-run heel horn exposes sensitive laminae
- contralateral claw: check for similar changes!
- at typical site (see Definition) granulation tissue may protrude through undermined horn
- under-running commonly extends cranially and peripherally to abaxial white line

Bacteriology: none in primary condition.

Pathology: horn defect originates from damaged pododerm, which may be secondary result of laminitis (coriosis, *pododermatitis aseptica diffusa*), poor trimming, and heel horn deformity. Caudal border of distal phalanx and insertion of deep digital flexor tendon (see Figure 7.4) both lie below typical site and are involved in complicated cases (see Section 7.11, p. 219 on deep digital sepsis).

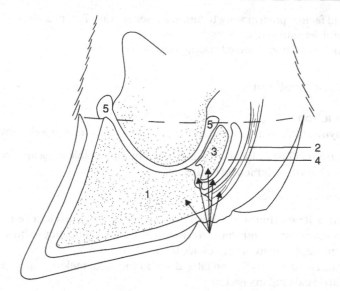

Figure 7.4 Typical site of sole ulcer of lateral hind claw with adjacent structures that may be affected by deep sepsis: 1. distal phalanx; 2. deep digital flexor tendon; 3. distal sesamoid (navicular bone); 4. navicular bursa; 5. distal interphalangeal joint.

Differential diagnosis: solear abscessation due to foreign body penetration, aseptic pododermatitis (solear haemorrhage) elsewhere in weight-bearing surface, simple heel erosion, subacute laminitis.

Treatment
- trim all feet initially or at end
- IVRA (intravenous regional analgesia, see Section 1.8, p. 33)
- remove under-run horn, trim horn of wall and heel so that weight-bearing by affected claw is minimal
- possibly apply block (hoof resin) to sound claw which should be minimally trimmed, if weight-bearing cannot otherwise be reduced
- remove protruding granulation tissue, leaving healthy pododerm and apply tetracycline spray, and bandage (waterproof) for five days
- alternatively, put on sulphadimidine powder, bandage (Vetrap®), and spray oxytetracycline over bandage to prevent wicking by mud into bandage
- broad spectrum antibiotics in septic cases
- confine to box and straw bedding for five days

Prophylaxis
- avoid overgrown claws by emphasising need for routine trimming (see Section 7.14, p. 232)

- avoid factors predisposing to laminitis (see Section 7.9, p. 210) and inter-digital dermatitis (e.g. excessive moisture)
- do not breed from affected young cows

7.7 Punctured sole

Introduction

Synonym: *pododermatitis septica (traumatica)*, septic (traumatic) pododermatitis.

Definition: diffuse or localised septic inflammation of solear corium, causing moderate to severe lameness if purulent.

Incidence: sporadic.

Predisposition: thin solear horn from preceding laminitis (coriosis) excessive abrasion from rough concrete, rough tracks, any tendency to hustle herd along inside passageways or outside tracks.

Corium (pododerm) has no fatty tissue in toe area, making entry of infection into distal phalanx easier.

Signs
- sudden onset of lameness (LS 2), usually in hindlimb, with solear penetration
- site often near toe or adjacent to white line
- defect in horn extends to solear pododerm, with variable under-running and pus production (black colour)
- localised pain

Aetiology: often iatrogenic following removal of excessive horn during trimming; also see Predisposition above. Foreign bodies (FB) include stones, often flints, nails, wire and thorns.

Bacteriology: secondary infection often mixed, including *Arcanobacterium pyogenes*.

Pathology: see Definition; Secondary complication is osteomyelitis of distal phalanx or distal interphalangeal joint (see Figure 7.4).

Differential diagnosis: subacute laminitis, solear ulceration, toe ulcer interdigital necrobacillosis.

Treatment
- primarily surgical: identify and remove FB; drain after exposure of under-run horn
- local astringent dressing
- curette distal phalanx if involved
- possibly elevate sole by block on other digit

- single injection of long-acting oxytetracycline if soft tissue (corium) is severely damaged
- tetanus prophylaxis indicated in known tetanus environment

Prophylaxis
- avoid predisposing causes contributing to poor quality of solear horn, i.e. laminitis (coriosis)
- good hygiene (foreign body disposal)
- if track to pasture is hazardous due to flints, consider installation of 'friendly' cow track

7.8 White line separation and abscessation

Introduction
Synonym: white line disease.

Definition: abaxial, or less commonly axial, wall separation from laminae at sole-wall area extending proximally, with cavity impacted with mud, faeces; or with development of abscess cavity at deepest part (abscessation).

Incidence: high and in some areas is major cause of digital lameness.

Predisposition and pathogenesis:
- abnormal horn production resulting from laminitic insult (coriosis)
- insufficient hoof trimming
- related to peripartum events some months previously

Signs
- moderate lameness (LS 1–2)
- white line wider than usual, and in early stages has series of pinpoint dark marks, later obvious foreign material impacted in white line
- separation evident on paring, no pain
- cases of white line abscessation are lame and have pain localised to wall
- internal wall abscess, without obvious track distally, also very sensitive to pincers pressure
- advanced cases have supracoronary septic sinus discharge (see Section 7.11, p. 219)

Aetiology: see **Predisposition**.

Bacteriology: *Arcanobacterium pyogenes* in abscessation.

Pathology: pressure necrosis of wall laminae, possibly also of solear laminae, following under-running and septic laminitis tracking progressively more proximally after entry of purulent micro-organisms, with absence of natural drainage distally due to impacted material.

Differential diagnosis: solear foreign body, laminitis, small coronary sandcrack.

Treatment

- routine trimming of all digits
- pare off wall over impacted and septic area to achieve drainage and prevent further impaction
- also remove all under-run sole (some cases have a large 'false sole')
- apply local antiseptic dressing (e.g. oxytetracycline spray) and firm dressing
- pare horn to normal shape of claw
- consider block on ipsilateral claw
- in septic cases give broad spectrum antibiotics for three days

Radical surgery, possibly amputation, is required in involvement of coronary tissues and distal interphalangeal joint (see Sections 7.11 and 7.12, pp. 219–225).

Prophylaxis

Avoid predisposing factors for laminitis (coriosis) (see Section 7.9 below), and ensure regular hoof trimming.

7.9 Laminitis (coriosis)

Introduction

Synonym: *Pododermatitis aseptica diffusa*, coriosis, 'founder'.

Definition: diffuse acute, subacute, subclinical or chronic inflammation of pododerm, usually in several digits. Chronic cases without acute stage (subclinical) are often seen.

Incidence: sporadic acute cases, widespread subacute, subclinical and chronic cases commonly in dairy units, high incidence in recently calved heifers and younger cows around parturition. Acute form occasionally presents as outbreak in barley beef units. Common in beef feedlots.

Predisposition:

- inherited factors (proven in Jersey)
- parturition
- feeding stress (ruminal lactic acidosis, subacute ruminal acidosis or SARA) from change of dry cow concentrate diet to high production rations, with potentially dangerous reduction of roughage intake
- exacerbation by trauma (overburdening), as in excessive standing due to reluctance to use cubicles (inexperience, bullying by herdmates)

Signs

- acute stage: painful hot digit, digital arterial pulsation, general depression, severe lameness, abnormal stance, possibly recumbent (LS 2–3)
- subacute: less painful but persistent stiffness, stilted gait, solear and white line haemorrhages (LS 1)
- chronic: stiff gait or not lame (LS 0–1), 'slipper foot' malformation with horizontal lines on wall, concave dorsal wall, widened white line and evidence of old solear amd white line haemorrhages. See section on pathology below

Aetiology: see Predisposition and Pathology.

Bacteriology: none.

Pathology: blood and serum exudation in acute stage, later (chronic) grooves on hoof wall, concave profile, widened white line and flat sole. Significant sinking of distal phalax due to peripartum slackening of the connective tissue support structures has been proved; thin sole or ulceration near tip of distal phalanx ('toe ulcer') is evident as haemorrhage ('bruising') as toe tip has no fat layer in its corium. White line lesions may develop into white line disease (see Section 7.8, p. 209); sole lesions at sole-heel junction may develop into solear ulceration (see Section 7.6, p. 206).

Histopathology: oedema, haemorrhages and thrombosis in acute stage, fibrosis and chronic thrombosis in later stages.

Differential diagnosis: bruised sole, white line disease, punctured sole, solear ulceration all of which may be present (see Figure 7.2).

Treatment

- acute stage: give systemic NSAIDs (flunixine meglumine or meloxicam) or possibly corticosteroids (only if non-pregnant) and diuretics
- ensure exercise (to improve local circulation and further reduce developing oedema), preferably by turning on to soft ground, e.g. field
- remove any precipitating dietary causes
- feed no concentrates until acute phase is over
- in recumbent case consider digital nerve block to get heifer or cow to stand, then forced exercise
- subacute stage: as in acute case
- chronic case: hoof trimming

Prophylaxis

- avoid large amounts of prepartum concentrates ('steaming up' 'lead feeding'), which should not exceed 2 kg daily
- avoid high intake of concentrate in early lactation, and aim at peak yield about six weeks postpartum

- ensure ready access to roughage immediately before and after concentrate intake, or consider change to complete diet feeding (TMR, total mixed rations) if problem persists
- improve buffering capacity of rumen fluid (avoid lactic acidosis or SARA) by increasing saliva production: give iodide or rock salt, grass or lucerne nuts in concentrate
- consider adding 1% sodium bicarbonate to concentrate ration, which should be fed as three to four daily portions
- accustom down-calving heifers gradually to concrete yards and cubicles several weeks beforehand, but ensure plenty of exercise in both pre- and post-partum weeks
- avoid exposure to excessive sole wear from long stony tracks, rough concrete
- high fibre diets should be used in rearing dairy heifers in long term planning
- ensure regular claw examination and trimming

Discussion
Excess lactic acid production alters rumenal bacterial flora, and causes release of bacterial endotoxins involving histamine release and stagnation of blood in laminae of digital horn, with consequent hypoxia and functional ischaemia. Ischaemic necrosis of the corium and laminae heals by fibrosis. These tissues then inevitably produce defective (soft, poor quality) horn in aberrant manner, resulting in signs seen in subacute and chronic stages. Toxic conditions (mastitis, metritis) may also contribute to development of laminitis in some dairy cattle.

7.10 Other digital conditions

(a) Digital dermatitis (Mortellaro)

Introduction
Synonym: *dermatitis digitalis*, 'hairy warts', PDD, papillomatous dermatitis.

Definition: circumscribed superficial ulceration of skin bordering coronary margin at heels, occasionally more dorsally. Can develop into mass of verrucose fronds (see Verrucose dermatitis, p. 214).

Incidence: Widespread in many dairy farms in western Europe (UK, Netherlands, Germany, etc.) and North America (California, New York State, etc.), where incidence can reach 100% and prevalence 20%. Often the major lameness problem.

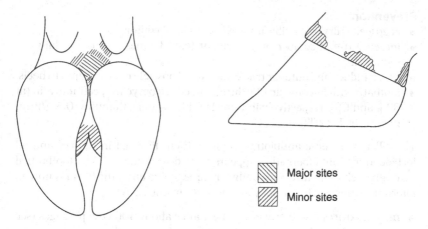

Major sites

Minor sites

Figure 7.5 Major and minor sites of digital dermatitis.

Signs
- predisposition is not known, but disease affects adult cattle causing variable and often severe lameness (LS 1–3)
- white epithelial border and signs of surrounding chronic dermatitis
- caudally in skin adjacent to heel horn, also occasionally anterior interdigital space, coronary band or in granulation tissue on sole (see Figure 7.5)
- apparently contagious, mostly introduced into 'clean' farm by bought-in heifers which may not themselves show clinical lesions
- role of skin microtrauma as permitting entry of organisms is speculative.

Bacteriology: believed to involve a *Treponema* genus spirochaete, possibly also a longer filamentous organism. Other postulated organisms include *Borrelia burgdorferi, Dichelobacter nodosus* and *Campylobacter* spp.

Differential diagnosis: possibly interdigital dermatitis, heel horn erosion, plantar eczema, but lesions are usually unmistakable.

Treatment
- treat all but most severe lesions in milking parlour
- cleanse with water spray, wait one minute, and apply topical aerosol antibiotic, e.g. oxytetracycline, daily for three days (long angled nozzle facilitates spray direction)
- drugs have included oxytetracycline, lincomycin, erythromycin and lincomycin/spectinomycin, and tylosin
- severe proliferating masses ('hairy warts') should be resected through epidermis (not subcutis) under local anaesthesia (e.g. IVRA, see Section 1.8, p. 35) in crush/chute.

Prevention
- keep feet as dry as possible improving cubicle bedding
- increase use of scraper or equivalent (e.g. 3 times, not twice daily) to reduce slurry
- check indoor and outdoor tracks for sites of possible microtrauma to heels
- footbath with lincomycin (1 g/litre), mixed lincomycin/spectinomycin (at 33 g and 66 g respectively in total 150 litre water), tiamulin (0.5 g/litre) or tylosin (1.2 g/litre).

The efficacy of these antibiotics (none of them licensed in the UK and all forbidden in Dutch footbaths) appears to be decreasing: initially footbathed through such a mixture once daily for three to five days, the trend is now to alternate drugs and to use daily for a minimum one week.

- most mixtures lose therapeutic effect after about 300 cow passages (see Section 7.15, p. 234)
- various other chemical mixtures have also been used with variable results
- isolate any newly purchased heifers for three weeks and check for overt digital dermatitis lesions, and treat or cull if affected
- disinfect all foot paring instruments (knives, clippers, crush/chute) after working with an infected herd

(b) Verrucose dermatitis

Introduction
Synonyms: *dermatitis verrucosa*, heel warts, 'hairy warts'.

Definition: moist proliferation of the dorsal and/or plantar/palmar skin, later developing wart-like proliferations, a common form of digital dermatitis (see Section 7.10a, p. 212) especially in parts of USA (CA, NY).
Microbiology is similar to the more ulcerative type seen commonly in Europe.

Signs treatment and prophylaxis: see Digital dermatitis p. 212. Histopathologically the lesion mass appears to be a papilloma.

(c) Interdigital dermatitis

Introduction
Synonyms: *dermatitis interdigitalis*.

Definition: inflammation of interdigital skin without extension to deeper tissues, and variable associated disturbance of horn growth.

Incidence and predisposition: widespread in certain moist housing systems and wet climates, in all age groups.

Signs
- mild inflammatory lesions of interdigital skin causing little or no lameness (LS 0–1)
- bulb horn clefts can lead to contusion of corium and sometimes eventually to solear ulceration. Lameness may be severe and chronic in such cases.

Aetiology: chronic mild irritation in moist conditions where bacterial infection is important and significant.

Bacteriology: *Dichelobacter nodosus* consistently recovered in some areas. *Fusobacterium necrophorum* also present.

Pathology: dermatitis characterised by polymorphonuclear cell infiltration of dermal structures damaged by associated bacterial invasion of germinal layer.

Hyperkeratosis and parakeratosis can follow. Disintegration of epidermis may spread to heel horn with contusion of corium and secondary ulceration.

Differential diagnosis: interdigital necrobacillosis, heel erosion, digital dermatitis.

Treatment
- pare off any diseased horn
- single severe case: interdigital spray with oxytetracycline or copper sulphate
- multiple cases: formalin or copper sulphate footbath (see Section 7.15, pp. 234–235)
- regular foot paring
- put into dry housing and dry grazing
- consider formalin footbath for herd control

Prophylaxis
Dry housing and grazing, regular footbaths and foot paring.

Discussion
Interdigital dermatitis has low incidence in UK, despite frequency of heel erosion (see below). *D. nodosus* has (1985) been recovered from typical lesions in the USA.

Relationship of interdigital dermatitis to digital dermatitis is hotly disputed.

(d) Heel erosion ('slurry heel')

Introduction
Synonym: *erosio ungulae*.

Definition: irregular loss of bulbar horn in form of multiple blackish pit or pock-like depressions or later deeper oblique grooves, usually affecting hind digits more severely than fore.

Incidence: widespread in winter-housed cattle from yearlings to adults, usually disappears at grass.

Predisposition: wet environment, long-term exposure to slurry, possible sequel to interdigital dermatitis, unrelated to parturition.

Signs

Slight or no lameness (LS 0–1) except in deep chronic cleft formation, which may damage corium, cause mild lameness, and lead to under-run heel.

Aetiology: chronic irritation, bacterial infection, interdigital dermatitis.

Bacteriology: *Dichelobacter nodosus* and *Fusobacterium necrophorum*.

Pathology: imperfect horn production and destruction. Corium traumatised by exposure to contusion on edges of clefts. Loss of much heel horn allows foot to rotate backwards and predisposes claw to sole ulcer as pedal bone increasingly compresses corium at 'typical site'.

Differential diagnosis: interdigital dermatitis.

Treatment

- single case: pare away diseased and under-run horn, spray topical oxytetracycline gentian violet aerosol on to any exposed corium and transfer to dry floor
- multiple cases: foot paring, footbaths (formalin) at twice weekly intervals
- if feasible, transfer to dry environment
- if not feasible, put lime into cubicles to disinfect and dry out heel horn

(e) Longitudinal (vertical) or transverse (horizontal) sandcrack or fissure

Introduction

Synonym: *fissura ungulae longitudinalis et transversalis*.

Definition: fissure of horny wall parallel to dorsal wall or parallel to coronet. An uncommon form is an axial wall crack or fissure.

Incidence: low in dairy breeds, but high incidence (prevalence 37%) found in some Hereford beef cows in Canada.

Predisposition: transverse form predisposed by overgrowth of digital horn and severe chronic laminitic horn rings (hardship lines or grooves). Longitudinal form predisposed by dry environment, trauma at coronary band.

Signs

- transverse form usually cosmetic blemish only, no lameness

- single claw form indicates local stress; multiple claws (e.g. all eight) indicates systemic insult e.g. parturition, diet change, altered environment
- pododerm rarely exposed
- longitudinal form may be gross and involve whole length of coronet to bearing surface
- in other longitudinal cases diagnosis is difficult when fissure is limited to small and extremely painful coronary lesion, which is partly obscured by hairs. Such cases have severe trauma to pododerm and early entry of infection.
- axial wall fissure is also hard to identify and can extend to coronary band causing severe pain

Aetiology: see Predisposition.

Bacteriology: no role in primary lesion.

Pathology: see above.

Differential diagnosis: transverse form – none. Longitudinal form – often missed at initial superficial examination of muddy claw. Distinguish interdigital necrobacillosis and punctured sole.

Treatment
- transverse form: pare distal section of horn, especially when it forms hinge with more proximal portion and can cause pain on underlying laminae when flexed upwards: shorten toe and bearing surface to avoid movement of fractured portion
- longitudinal form: remove any excessive granulation tissue (pododerm) protruding through sandcrack
- cleanse well, local astringent, local antibiotic spray, bandage and rest, possibly with block on adjacent claw especially with painful involvement of coronary band
- in severe case clean fissure well with grinder or Dremel drill, drill hole at proximal end of crack and fill with resin, and block other digit

Guarded prognosis in vertical fissures.

Prophylaxis
Regular foot trimming, use of oils on at-risk cattle in dry environment.

(f) Fracture of distal phalanx (pedal bone)

Introduction
Unless involving pathological fracture (as in osteomyelitis, see Toe Ulcer p. 208) this fracture is almost invariably intra-articular (see Figure 7.6).

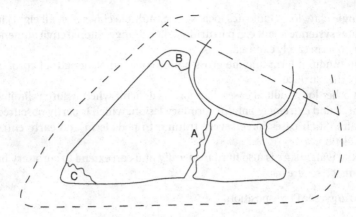

Figure 7.6 Common sites of distal phalangeal (pedal bone) fractures:
A. intra-articular to distal surface; B. occasionally involving extensor process;
C. tip of distal phalanx, often secondary pathological fracture following toe ulcer and osteomyelitis.

Incidence: uncommon, usually in one to five year olds, no breed prevalence. Associated with trauma such as bulling activity in a concrete yard or following first turnout into a rock-hard pasture, broken slatted floors, fluorosis, subclinical osteoporosis, and pathological fractures in osteomyelitis.

Signs
- sudden onset lameness (usually medial claw) in fore leg (LS 3), occasionally hind leg
- rarely bilateral
- medial digit of forelimb commonly involved; limb is typically carried across midline of body to minimise weight-bearing; occasionally cross-legged stance or leg held forward in stall or cubicle
- no digital swelling, possibly slight heat
- pain on percussion, or pincer pressure and extension (see Figure 7.6)
- flexion of digit resented
- diagnosis on medio-lateral radiograph of affected medial digit (plate inserted interdigitally), usually intra-articular

Differential diagnosis: acute laminitis, foreign body penetration, bilateral foreclaw sole ulcers, acute interdigital necrobacillosis, infected vertical fissure of hoof wall.

Treatment
- untreated animals remain lame for many weeks, as intra-articular fracture heals slowly
- block sound hoof (see Section 7.26, pp. 255–257), resulting in immediate improvement and accelerating healing rate

- also useful to wire toe of affected digit in flexed position to wooden block on sound digit
- digital amputation rarely indicated

7.11 Deep digital sepsis

Development
Conditions described in preceding sections involve superficial structures (see Sections 7.5 and 7.10) and/or the sensitive pododerm (see Sections 7.6–7.9). Deep digital sepsis can result from the spread of several conditions, listed below:

Solear ulceration (see Figure 7.4):
- necrosis of deep flexor tendon (upward tilting of digit)
- osteomyelitis of distal phalanx and distal sesamoid
- septic navicular bursitis
- distal interphalangeal septic arthritis
- ascending septic tenosynovitis of common digital flexor sheath

Coriosis (laminitis) white line sepsis, punctured sole:
- solear abscessation
- osteomyelitis of distal phalanx and septic navicular bursitis
- distal interphalangeal septic arthritis
- septic spread to coronet, possibly partial or total secondary exungulation

Toe ulcer:
- distal phalangeal osteitis

Interdigital necrobacillosis:
- distal interphalangeal septic arthritis
- septic tenosynovitis of digital flexor tendon sheath
- retro-articular abscess of bulb

Sandcrack (fissure) at coronary band (infected):
- distal interphalangeal joint
- distal sesamoidean (navicular) bursa
- common digital flexor tendon sheath
- surrounding soft tissues including retro-articular heel bulb

Organism of greatest importance is *Arcanobacterium pyogenes*. Ascending infection usually travels primarily via synovial fluid along digital flexor sheath, eventually infecting the fetlock joint by bursting through sheath. Fetlock joint capsule, common to all the fetlock articular surfaces, is large and mobile. The pastern joint capsule has limited capacity and is relatively less mobile, with no connection between the two digits.

Signs

Progressively severe lameness (LS 3), possibly leading to recumbency, pyaemia, weight loss, poor appetite, swelling and erythema around coronet and pastern, later involving flexor tendon sheath, and extensive distal limb oedema. Most cases develop a fistulous track.

Treatment

Medical and conservative surgical methods

Systemic antibiotics alone are most unlikely to control infection, since the blood supply does not extend to septic foci in the osteomyelitic bone or tendon sheath, and the antibiotic fails to penetrate these infected areas.

Conservative methods include:

- application of cast (fibreglass, resin etc). The aim is to permit infection to be walled off by fibrosis, with eventual development of ankylosis of septic joint. The technique is simple. The disadvantages are prolonged disease course, considerable pain and discomfort, and risk of pyaemia, death or cull, with condemnation of carcass
- conservative surgical drainage and irrigation of septic foci. The advantage is preservation of the digit. Several disadvantages in chronic cases include: need for good anatomical knowledge, several visits and possibly daily irrigation, it is expensive, and eventually may fail due to spread
- surgical drainage and irrigation with curettage, often leading to facilitated ankylosis

Advantages and disadvantages are as for preceding technique, but there is less risk of failure from spread.

Radical surgical techniques

These involve resection of diseased structures:

- amputation of digit (see Section 7.12 below)
- resection of distal sesamoidean part of deep flexor tendon (see Section 7.13, p. 225)
- resection of deep flexor tendon from site proximal to fetlock joint (see Section 7.13, p. 226).

7.12 Digital amputation

Indications

Indications, in descending order of frequency are:

- septic arthritis of distal interphalangeal joint
- septic tenosynovitis of deep flexor

- osteomyelitis of distal sesamoid
- osteomyelitis of distal phalanx
- severe digital trauma, e.g. exungulation, loss of much coronary band
- sepsis of coronary band and supracoronary soft tissues.

Frequently several of the above indications are present.

Advantages

- immediate removal of potentially lethal material (reducing risk of pyaemic spread)
- relief of pain
- relatively rapid return to thriftiness and production with improved condition and milk yield
- simple surgical technique compared with alternatives

Disadvantages

- potential failure if case selection is poor and infection is present above amputation site
- persisting poor gait in some heavy cows and bulls due to altered stance and strain on remaining digit, especially in difficult terrain
- lowered market value
- few cows with amputated digits are retained for more than eighteen months

Technique

Sedate animal (xylazine 0.1–0.2 mg/kg i.m. or acepromazine 0.1 mg/kg i.m.) and cast with affected digit uppermost (often lateral hind), or work with cow standing in Wopa crush (see p. 35). Produce suitable analgesia by:

- intravenous regional analgesia (IVRA) (see Section 1.8, p. 33) which is preferred method, or ring block above fetlock
- examine digits to check that infection has not reached level of fetlock joint, and that sepsis is confined to distal part of proximal phalanx and more distal structures
- clip hair from level of fetlock distally to coronet over affected side and over median line, i.e. interdigital space
- remove caked faeces, use stiff brush, run bandage through interdigital space, and give surgical scrub to area

Amputation through distal third of proximal phalanx

Method of amputation obliquely through distal third of proximal phalanx (see Figure 7.7), without preservation of skin flap, is preferred method:

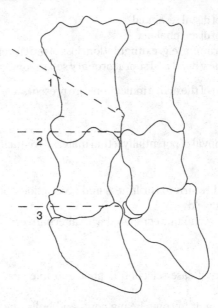

Figure 7.7 Sites for digital amputation or disarticulation.
1. amputation with oblique cut in distal third of proximal phalanx (open or skin flap technique both possible); 2. exarticulation through proximal interphalangeal joint; 3. exarticulation through distal interphalangeal joint.

- apply tourniquet above fetlock or hock, if not already in position for IVRA
- incise interdigital space close to affected digit along whole length, continuing proximally 3 cm dorsally, and 2.5 cm at plantar aspect
- insert embryotomy (obstetrical) wire into incision and adjust to a level 1–2 cm above axial aspect of proximal interphalangeal joint
- with assistant firmly holding digit down towards ground, saw rapidly at an oblique angle so that cut emerges 2–3 cm above abaxial joint level, continuing through skin
- trim off protruding interdigital fat pad
- twist off any major vessels e.g. dorsal digital artery lying axially
- examine cut surface meticulously for signs of s.c. abscessation and necrosis, peritendinous infection and septic tenosynovitis
- massage distally along deep flexor tendon sheath to check synovia (see Table 7.1)
- purulent synovia should be irrigated out of tendon sheath (male dog catheter, 50 ml syringe and saline), and reconsider need for resection of part of deep flexor tendon
- dress wound with oxytetracycline or sulphadimidine powder (not essential), apply gauze swab or paraffin-impregnated tulle, and hold in place by

Table 7.1 Some characteristics of normal and pathological synovia.

Diagnosis	Turbidity	Clotting	WBC ×10⁹/l	%N	Protein (g/l)	Mucin precipitate
Normal	0	0	<0.25	<10	<1.5	tight, ropy
Septic or suspect septic	+++	+++	>20	80	>3	very abnormal
Aseptic	+	variable	3	<30	<3	abnormal
Osteoarthritis (degenerative)	0 or +	0	<0.2	<10	<3	normal or almost normal
Hydrops	0 or +	0	<0.35	<10	<2	normal

0 = negative; +, ++ and +++ indicate increasing degrees of severity, N = Neutrophils; WBC = White bloodcells

pressure bandage and possibly protect by waterproof covering (e.g. duct tape)
- in bandaging avoid pressure necrosis around accessory digits
- remove tourniquet
- inject single prophylactic dose of ceftiofur or long-acting oxytetracycline and, in known risk areas, tetanus antitoxin

Aftercare
- change dressing after two days, when cut surface should be cleaned and checked for residual infection
- foul odour suspicious
- apply new dressing for six days
- surface may then safely be left exposed for granulation and epithelialisation
- rinse wound with water once daily until healing well

Animal should be kept in dry surroundings, either housed (preferably) or outdoors on dry level ground, during the three week recovery period.

Alternative amputation techniques
(see Figure 7.7)

Exarticulation at proximal interphalangeal joint
Advantages are:

- end result of surgery is hollow cavity ideal for pressure packing by bandage or swabs
- avoids exposure of medullary cavity of proximal phalanx which could allegedly become focus of post-operative infection

Disadvantages:

- lengthy procedure
- difficult to locate joint level axially for incision to expose articulation
- liability to break scalpel blades in this awkward site
- preferable use of 'sage knife' (a curved solid two-edged instrument) and a small curette

Amputation through coronary band

Involves subsequent removal of extensor process of distal phalanx, proximal part of middle phalanx and the distal sesamoid.

This technique is laborious, but was developed to retain potential for growth of a weight-bearing horny wall after surgery. Surgery preferably in recumbent patient.

- groove is made 1 cm distal to horn-skin margin of coronary band
- obstetrical wire saw cut to remove claw, passing through distal interphalangeal joint
- removal of extensor process of distal phalanx, transecting extensor tendon at insertion
- removal of proximal part of middle phalanx and distal sesamoid
- curettage of distal articular cartilage of proximal phalanx
- sharp dissection of any septic or otherwise discoloured soft tissue, or radical curettage

Skin flap preservation

Skin flap may be preserved and placed over amputation surface, following removal of digit through distal one third of proximal phalanx. Advantage is cosmetic improvement and faster healing.

Disadvantages include:

- inability to inspect amputation site when dressing is changed
- suture tear out due to post-operative swelling
- risk of skin necrosis
- good case selection is essential (no phlegmon present)

Skin flap is created initially by semicircular incision from 5–6 cm above interdigital space on dorsal and plantar aspects, passing down to the coronary band. Ensure this flap is large and thick, and is then reflected proximally. Amputation is done in conventional way and skin flap, trimmed as needed, is then sutured over stump.

Discussion

Average survival period following digital amputation in commercial dairy herds ranges from 12–24 months. Exceptions survive for years. Eventual reason for disposal is further digital disease in over half of these cattle. In majority of cases digital amputation has no effect on yield in the lactation subsequent to the one in which amputation is performed.

Amputation of accessory digits ('dewclaws')

Indication
Prophylactic surgery on medial accessory digits of hindlimbs to prevent self-inflicted teat trauma. Ethical as well as scientific objections to technique in Europe, therefore forbidden in many countries including UK and Switzerland. Common routine procedure in many North American dairies.

Technique
- remove at two to eight weeks old in recumbent calf
- clean and disinfect area
- local infiltration analgesia (2 ml 2% lignocaine plain)
- push digit proximally to move away from joint space and major vessels
- resect through skin margin and dewclaw base with large scissors or Barnes dehorner, remaining superficial and so avoiding deeper digital vasculature
- suture any wounds with significant haemorrhage
- apply topical antibacterial powder, dry swab and adhesive tape dressing for one week

7.13 Other digital surgery

(a) Resection of digital flexor tendon and their sheaths following digital amputation

Indication
Extension of infection above level of proposed amputation, without involvement of fetlock joint, is indication for resection of part of deep and superficial flexor tendons and their sheaths.

Treatment

Resection of superficial and deep flexor tendon after amputation
- identify common digital flexor tendon sheath, and insert straight metal probe proximally about 6 cm
- incise through skin, tendon sheath and part of annular ligament down to superficial flexor tendon
- remove superficial and deep tendon by cutting transversely at proximal point
- remove any exposed, purulent or necrotic sheath
- dress wound and leave to heal by granulation tissue
- alternatively, suture skin only

Alternative method, using approach above fetlock
- incise skin 3 cm proximal to accessory digit immediately over proximal border of flexor digital sheath
- continue this vertical incision down to superficial flexor tendon
- transect both flexor tendons at this point and pull out tendon from amputation site
- remove any septic areas of sheath, which are less well exposed in this method

(b) Resection of deep and superficial flexor tendons and sheaths (see Figure 7.8)

Indication
Septic tenosynovitis complicating deep digital sepsis.

Treatment
Sometimes removal of deep digital tendon is adequate. Other possible procedures are removal of deep and superficial tendons with or without partial or total removal of digital sheath. Precise procedure depends on extent of sepsis at surgical investigation.

Technique
- useful instruments include a blunt-ended curved tenotome and long slightly curved scissors
- tourniquet at mid-metatarsal (-carpal) region and IVRA (see Section 1.8, pp. 33–36)
- trim back accessory claws
- surgical skin preparation to mid-metatarsus (-carpus)
- skin, subcutis and horn of heel bulb are incised over deep flexor tendon from affected distal area (e.g. sole-heel junction), keeping incision axial to accessory digit to point 5 cm proximal to fetlock joint
- open sheath along plantar (volar) aspect
- cut through superficial flexor tendon longitudinally over fetlock (where it encloses deep flexor)
- section deep flexor transversely, just distal to bifurcation (5 cm proximal to fetlock)
- retract tendon from incision and transect distally at insertion into distal phalanx
- check any severe involvement of superficial tendon and, if necessary, resect proximally at same level as deep flexor and at insertion to middle phalanx
- dissect free and resect any infected tendon sheath and areas of subcutaneous abscessation including curettage as required

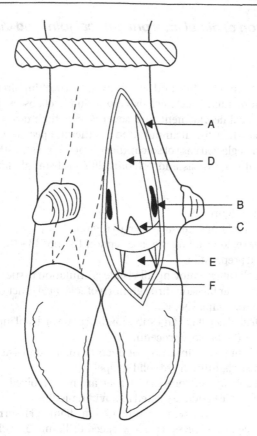

Figure 7.8 Surgical anatomy for removal of superficial and deep digital flexor tendons following proximal spread of deep infection.
A. incision 12 cm long from proximal to fetlock distally into heel horn; B. sectioned fetlock ligament; C. opened common digital sheath; D. superficial flexor tendon; E. deep digital flexor tendon; F. distal cruciate ligament superficial to distal sesamoid and distal interphalangeal joint.

- note that minimal amount of tissue should be resected
- dress wound with povidine-iodine-soaked gauze, pack wound, and close proximal half (to below dewclaws) with simple interrupted skin sutures
- keep wound open distally for drainage and removal of gauze packing; bandage firmly
- apply block to sound claw, and wire toes together
- systemic antibiotics for seven to ten days
- change dressing at two, seven and fourteen days, or more frequently if necessary

(c) Resection of distal interphalangeal joint and distal sesamoid

Indications
Purulent infection of joint and osteomyelitis resulting from spread of solear ulceration, interdigital necrobacillosis and heel abscess in cases non-responsive to local débridement and several days high dosage of systemic antibiotics, and when digital amputation is either not permitted or desirable. Typically it is a neglected case of solear ulceration (abscess) with severe distal interphalangeal joint sepsis and osteomyelitis of distal phalanx and distal sesamoid.

Technique (see Figure 7.9)
- tourniquet at mid-metatarsal (-carpal) region
- intravenous regional analgesia (see Section 1.8, pp. 33–36)
- surgical skin preparation
- carefully probe after removing all visible granulation tissue
- 3–3.5 cm circular incision through horn of sole-heel junction
- remove distal sesamoid bone
- drill out infected cartilage and subchondral bone of distal interphalangeal joint surfaces ('apple core procedure')
- resect any remains of insertion of deep flexor tendon with 'sage' knife (double-sided, slightly curved solid scalpel)
- if skin and subcutis of coronary border are not involved in sepsis, pack cavity with sterile bandage soaked in povidine-iodine
- if coronet is involved, remove skin (2 cm diameter) surrounding any fistula or incipient abscess with low speed drill, make track 0.8–1.2 cm diameter from sole up through coronary defect
- evaluate usefulness of irrigation tube into cavity and fixed along metatarsus
- insert bandage as above (unless twice daily irrigation is planned)
- put block on sound digit
- wire toes to prevent over-extension of operated digit
- high dosage of systemic antibiotics for ten days
- change dressing at two days, then weekly intervals, until granulation tissue has filled defect
- remove block and wire at six to twelve weeks

Intensive post-operative care is essential. If infection spreads nevertheless, digital amputation may be only alternative to cull (carcass condemnation due to antibiotic residues!)

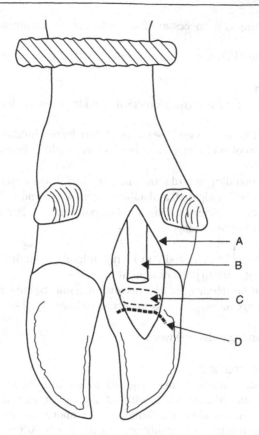

Figure 7.9 Resection of distal interphalangeal joint in deep digital sepsis (right hind lateral).
A. plantar skin incision (compare Figure 7.8); B. deep digital flexor tendon, resected distal portion; C. distal sesamoid; D. plantar margin of distal interphalangeal joint.

(d) Removal of interdigital hyperplastic skin (see Section 7.5)

Methods include knife surgery, electrocautery and cryosurgery (see Section 1.14, p. 49).

Technique
- give sedative (xylazine or acepromazine, see Section 1.6, pp. 13–16 and Section 7.15, pp. 204–205)
- restrain in crush/chute (e.g. Wopa crate, see Section 1.8, pp. 35–36)
- IVRA, ring block or local infiltration (poor analgesia)
- cleanse area thoroughly, clip and disinfect

- apply tourniquet (unnecessary for cryosurgery) if not already in place for IVRA
- assistant should separate digits manually with length of bandage

Knife method
- grasp mass with Allis tissue forceps or Backhaus towel clamp (see Figure 1.1)
- remove whole mass in wedge-shaped pattern by two incisions
- keep fine lip of skin along axial borders from which re-epithelialisation will start
- remove protruding interdigital fat, avoiding distal cruciate ligaments (which are easily palpated) and adjacent coronary band
- apply oxytetracycline or sulphadimidine powder, interdigital pressure pad and figure of eight bandage
- release tourniquet
- wire toes together, especially in heavy animals, with drill holes 2.5 cm behind point of toe to prevent separation
- no systemic antibiotics, but tetanus antitoxin may be indicated
- do not change bandage unless site becomes infected, or bandage is blood-soaked
- remove bandage after one week

Electrocautery method
Although a hot iron may be used, the instrument must be small and precise to reach the interdigital mass without damaging surrounding tissues. Apply electrocautery loop as in knife surgery above, ensuring integrity of neighbouring structures especially cruciate ligaments. Advantage is reduced post-operative haemorrhage, disadvantage is slower healing. Toes should be wired together after dressing wound with powder

Cryosurgery method
Advantages include absence of haemorrhage and avoidance of post-operative bandaging and dressing.

- depending on size of lesion, some hyperplastic tissue may first be resected ('debulked') by knife
- apply probe to tissue to create ice ball (e.g. 3 cm diameter) in rapid freeze, followed by slow thaw cycle
- repeat at other sites, often totalling three, until whole area has been frozen once
- repeat freeze of each area once (with liquid nitrogen) or twice (N_2O or CO_2)
- do not bandage or dress the region. Wiring of toes contra-indicated
- mass will become necrotic in seven to ten days, and drop off a few days later leaving a granulating bed which will slowly epithelialise

Discussion

Recurrence is likely whichever technique is used. Consider foot conformation, possible inheritance, and trim claws at time of surgery and regularly thereafter. Recurrence rate may be reduced by keeping wire in place for one to two months

7.14 Hoof deformities, overgrowth and corrective foot trimming

Hoof deformities may be inherited, or acquired as a result of insufficient wear, or claw diseases such as laminitis. Studies by McDaniel (see Appendix 1, pp. 259–260), working on dairy cows in North Carolina, have been based on:

- length of dorsal hoof wall from coronet to toe (measured with pair of commercial dividers)
- angle of dorsal wall to ground (protractor)
- heel depth (pair of dividers) (see Figure 7.10)

It was found that:

- cows surviving for three or four lactations had shorter hooves and steeper angles than non-survivors, based on measurements made during the first lactation
- heritability of hoof length, employing sire comparisons, increased from first to fourth lactation
- increases in milk yield from first to second lactation were greater in cows with short, large-angled hooves in the first lactation

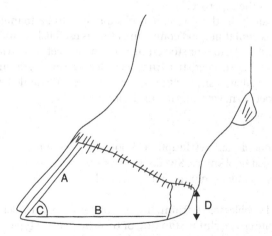

Figure 7.10 Diagram of vertical section through normal digit of adult dairy cow.
A. dorsal wall: length 75–80 mm (approximately 3 inches); B. bearing surface: length 130 mm (approximately 5 inches); C. dorsal wall angle: 50° forelimb, 55° hindlimb; D. heel height: 30–40 mm (approximately 1½ inches).

- first lactation cows with above features had shorter calving to conception interval following the second lactation
- high yielding cows tend to have longer and lower-angled hooves after their second parturition
- calving to conception interval within the same lactation was greater in cows with longer, smaller-angled hooves than in those with shorter, steeper-angled hooves.

Hoof traits of young cows are associated with their future economic worth. Since measurements were made from progeny of bulls high on milk yield, the variations of hoof traits are associated with survival rates, reproductive performance and increased yield from first to later lactations.

These facts emphasise the necessity to take corrective measures, including routine chiropody and to review breeding policy in herds where digital overgrowth is a major problem.

Corrective and preventative hoof trimming

Trimming is essential for the maintenance of healthy normal feet on most dairy farms as well as on artificial insemination centres where dozens of bulls are kept in confined conditions. Increasingly hoof trimming is being done well by full-time professional trimmers who have their own specialist equipment (e.g. purpose-built crushes/chutes, including the Wopa crate, or other models of turn-over devices, most mechanically powered). Trimmers often prefer to use powered metal disk grinders (angle grinders). Farm staff generally have insufficient time to deal with the feet of 150+ herd members and inevitably lack the expertise.

Since, certainly in the UK, foot problems tend to be managed by these trimmers, it is vital that good communication is established and maintained between trimmer, farmer or stock manager and the vet, who will be called in to treat cows where deeper structures are affected. Good written records (ID, lameness score, diagnosis, treatment, need for revisit) should be maintained for stockkeeper, farm veterinarian and trimmer.

Equipment
- single or double action (Hauptner) hoof pincers or 'nippers'
- right and left hoof knives, Swedish or German pattern
- rotary disk grinder (angle grinder, 10 cm disk)
- hoof rasp
- ropes and hobbles for restraint, hobbles preferably with Velcro® fastening
- appropriate crush/chute, standing or turn-over tilting type
- disinfectant bucket for instruments between cows
- protective goggles (horn particles and dust from grinder), possibly face mask, gloves and wrist protectors

- supply of prosthetic blocks and acrylic (Technovit®, Cowslip®, Shoof®, rubber block)

Timing of trimming
Ideally at drying off, and again, assuming twice yearly job, at winter housing or not later than one month before spring turnout but often done when time is available.

Site of trimming
- preferably under cover, but good light essential
- site should have easy route from collecting area and to outside yard for later inspection, and be easily cleansed

Technique (see Figure 7.11)
Standing behind a normal cow, an imaginary perpendicular line drawn through the hip joint should pass through the point of the hock and through the interdigital space. An abnormal stance of toe produces an inward turning of the hocks and outward pointing of the claws, indicating current or impending digital problems and lameness.

- check gait (possibly lameness score) and stance when going into crush
- raise hind limb, fix, and clean off mud and slurry with sawdust, straw or cloth (not water)
- start with minimal trim of medial claw using hoof pincers to shorten length with vertical cut ('dumping') to correct length or height (ideally 7.5 cm length of dorsal wall, but 8 cm acceptable in big-framed cows = length of cigarette packet) (see Figures 7.10, 7.1[1])

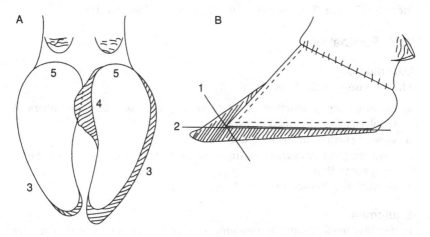

Figure 7.11 Steps in routine foot trimming of dairy cow with overgrown claws.

- effect is a square-ended toe 5–7 mm thick
- remove excess horn from sole surface near toe, correcting the square or stub toe appearance, and preserving heel horn [2]
- remove any excessive axial overlapping horn flap [3], [4]
- constantly check sole surface and white line, particularly abaxially, for haemorrhage or granulation tissue
- pare bearing surface slightly concave, with special attention to sole heel area but retain most heel horn [5]
- repeat technique on lateral claw, which almost invariably requires more attention
- continue with contralateral limb, and finally check forefeet
- lifting of forefeet seems more likely to lead to hindquarters collapse of cow, and is best prevented by belly band
- if sensitive corium is accidentally entered, and likely to result in lameness, consider putting block on ipsilateral claw

Discussion

Many dairy cows have grossly abnormal weight distribution of 70:30 on lateral and medial claws respectively. Recent (2003) studies on weight-bearing have shown that even after the above standard (Dutch method) trimming, balance has not been restored to the (theoretical) ideal of 50:50, but merely to 60:40. It is vital therefore that minimal amount of horn should be taken from medial claw.

Pare sole of lateral claw to same level as medial claw, and try to reduce heel depth to that of medial claw too.

Look at two heels from rear, or lay flat surface (e.g. hoof knife handle) transversely across heels to confirm their equal height

Ideal dorsal wall angle is 55° (hind) and 50° (forelimb). Ideal dorsal wall measures 7.5 cm (7–8 cm) from coronet to toe (see Figure 7.10).

7.15 Footbaths

Introduction

The purpose of footbaths is:

- inhibition or destruction of bacteria (e.g. *Fusobacterium necrophorum*) involved in interdigital skin diseases
- washing action, cleansing of digits
- hardening of sole horn, reducing wear rate and incidence of bruising and sole penetration
- control of digital dermatitis and heel erosion

Equipment

Preferably two footbaths, in tandem, with first containing water or a mild detergent mixture, the second the active solution.

Bath should be made of concrete (permanent), glass-reinforced concrete, or be a sheet-steel tray (portable). A tough sponge floor mat can much reduce the necessary fluid volume. Alternatively some straw is not only 'cow friendly' but tends to separate the claws so that fluid better soaks the interdigital cleft.

Dimensions of bath: minimum 3 m long; minimum 85 cm wide, depending on breed; 15–25 cm high, permitting fluid depth of 10–12 cm with non-slip floor.

Site the footbath in passageway or race at exit from milking parlour, preferably under cover, where dilution by rainwater can be avoided.

Bath fluid can be 2.5–5% formalin solution, alternatively 2.5% copper sulphate or zinc sulphate. Disadvantages exist. Formalin may irritate eyes and its disposal is viewed with suspicion by environmental health authorities e.g. UK Health and Safety Executive. Never exceed 5% formalin concentration, as 10% solution soon causes a severe localised chemical reaction and lameness. Ingested copper sulphate may cause acute copper poisoning.

Antibiotic footbaths for control of digital dermatitis: see Section 7.10a, p. 214.

The bath contents should be emptied into an appropriate collection facility, not to a watercourse or ground water.

Treatment

Ideally, stand lame cows (e.g. cases of interdigital necrobacillosis, interdigital or digital dermatitis, heel erosion and possibly solear ulceration) in bath for 20 minutes twice daily. This is rarely practical as it is too laborious on larger units today.

For preventative treatment walk cattle through after four successive milkings over a two-day period, then empty, clean and refill with water for five days. Repeat weekly throughout the year, except when frozen. Note that a standard bath is inactivated (i.e. bactericidal effect is lost) after 800 cow passages (e.g. 200 cows × 4 passages, viz. one week recommended usage). Recent Dutch studies suggest the figure of 800 should be reduced to 300.

Discussion

Regular formalin footbath usage should be practised in herds with an unacceptably high incidence of interdigital disease, heel erosion and solear ulceration. The lameness incidence will be reduced, and the severity of lesions will tend to be less, reducing further the economic losses.

7.16 Check lists for herd problems

Check lists for systemic and logical examination of herd digital lameness problem are useful aids. Tables 7.2–7.6 cover:

Table 7.2   Herd details: Name   Address   Reference   Vet/Trimmer.

1. Number of cows: milking _____
                    dry _____
                    total _____
2. Breed _____
3. Self contained or flying herd _____
4. AI or own bull(s), or both _____
5. Calving pattern (months) _____
6. Average yield (litres): cows _____
                            heifers _____
                            herd average _____
7. Current daily yield for herd: actual _____
                                 target _____
8. percentage of first calf heifers in herd _____
    percentage of second calf cows _____
    percentage of older (remaining) cows _____
9. Culling rate, as average of last two years: _____ individuals = _____
    Number of culls for: lameness _____
                         infertility _____
                         mastitis _____
                         mixed reasons, including lameness _____
                         other _____

Table 7.3   Description of lameness problem.

1. Are records of lame cows kept? Examine! _____
2. Total (or estimated) lame cows in last 12 months _____
    Total (or estimated) lame cows in preceding 12–24 month period _____
3. Total lameness treatments by farmer and vet in last 12 months _____
4. Maximum percentage of lame cows at any one time (prevalence) _____%
5. Dominant age group for lameness (first calf or second calvers
    or older cows) _____
6. Number of weeks before or after calving when most lameness
    cases appear _____
7. Forelimb or hindlimb problem _____
    Horn or soft tissue (skin) involvement _____
    Lateral or medial claw _____
8. Commonest diagnoses for lameness in last 12 months: digital
    dermatitis, interdigital necrobacillosis/solear bruising or
    penetration/solear ulceration/white line separation or
    abscessation/heel necrosis or separation under-running/other _____

Table 7.4 Herd investigation.

1. Prevalence of lameness today in milking herd
2. Conformation (for lame and sound cattle):
   Relative weight and size
   Size of digits
   Angle of hock (from lateral and caudal views)
   Outward angulation hind feet (°)
   Angle of dorsal wall (°)
   Height of heel
   Overgrowth of digits (nil, moderate, severe)
   Body score 1–5 (emaciated-fat)
3. Housing system:
   Cowshed/cubicles/straw yard
   Cowshed: size of standings
              surface characteristics (e.g. mats)
              bedding material
              exercise area
              passageway surface
              slats
              slurry quantity and quality
   Cubicles: cubicle size (length, width, step height)
              surface characteristics
   Concrete age and condition
   Doorways and passageways
   Overall cow concentration indoors (m² per cow)
   Distance travelled on cow tracks, surface and smoothness,
       roughness and wetness
4. Nutrition:
   Grazing, nature and conditions of herbage or crop
   Concentrate composition (% crude protein)
   Concentrate maximum intake (kg): before calving
                                    at peak yield
   Duration of steaming up (weeks)
   Period from calving to peak yield (weeks)
   Concentrate feeding: number of times per day where fed
   Roughage composition: % crude protein
                         % crude fibre
   Silage composition: % dry matter
                       acidity
                       palatability
   Roughage intake (kg dry matter):
              maximum intake before calving peak
              where fed
              whether fed with concentrates
   Supplements (salt, sodium bicarbonate, zinc, other):
              in concentrates
              fed separately

Continued

5. Prophylaxis:
   Foot-trimming: practice: none, self, visiting trimmer, vet _____
                     frequency/year _____
                     technique (e.g. grinder) _____
   Footbath: site _____
           composition _____
           concentration _____
           frequency of replenishment _____
           usage _____
   Quality of stockmanship (including weekend and holiday staff) _____

Table 7.5 Individual cow investigation.

1. Identification	_____
2. Number of calves bred	_____
Pregnancy (mo)/number of weeks postpartum	_____
Current yield/expected lactation yield (L)	_____
Current concentrate consumption (Kg)	_____
Body score 1–5 (emaciated-fat)	_____
3. Degree of lameness: severe/moderate/slight/non lame (3–0)	_____
Affected leg(s) LF RF LH RH	_____
Site: upper limb tissue primarily involved	_____
digit (interdigital or horn, lateral or medial claw)	_____
Estimated duration of lameness (weeks)	_____
Previous treatment (medical, surgical, trim)	_____
Diagnosis: major and/or minor	_____

- herd details
- description of lameness problem
- herd investigation
- individual cow investigation
- action recommendations

Numerous factors play interrelated roles in causing this 'production disease'. Investigation of herd problem should be done if lameness incidence exceeds 15–20%

7.17 Infectious arthritis ('joint ill') of calves

Introduction

Joint ill (neonatal polyarthritis) is usually caused by haematogenous spread of septic infection from the umbilicus, less commonly lungs or liver.

Table 7.6 Action recommendations.

1. Individual cow treatment:
   Surgical _____
   Medical _____
   Prophylactic (paring, footbath, etc) _____
2. Herd treatment and advice:
   Nutrition: alter amount and type of supplements? _____
              alter ratio of roughage to concentrate? _____
   Housing, e.g. give more exercising space _____
   Bedding, e.g. change bedding material _____
   Hygiene, e.g. scrape walkways and yards more often _____
   Foot-paring, trimming and technique _____
3. Further investigations:
   Feed analysis and amounts fed _____
   Examine and record more digits and limbs or more cows _____
   Investigate housed behaviour, walkways and pasture
     conditions _____
   Investigate footbath construction, solution and usage _____
   Investigate breeding records for familial predisposition _____
   Revisit in four weeks, three months re progress _____

Organisms may be *E. coli*, *Salmonella* spp. *Streptococcus* spp. and *Arcanobacterium pyogenes*, Major factors contributing to disease include the environmental pathogen load (i.e. cleanliness of parturition area) and the immune status of calf.

Signs
- depression, lameness or recumbency, anorexia, dehydration
- joint swelling and pain within 24 hours of onset of infection
- common sites include hock, stifle, carpus and fetlock (hip, shoulder rarely)
- umbilicus may show obvious signs of infection, with pain on deep palpation (see Section 3.13, p. 123 for routes of spread)
- later nervous signs (e.g. head tremors, opisthotonus) develop in some calves
- ancillary aids: arthrocentesis (cytology, culture!), radiography, ultrasound

Diagnosis
Swelling and pain in several joints (rarely with symmetrical involvement) in depressed calf are usually diagnostic

Treatment and prognosis
- cleanse umbilicus, consider removal later of septic umbilical focus
- systemic antibiotherapy e.g. ceftiofur for seven to ten days
- improve immune status with whole blood transfusion, other intravenous fluids

- immediate joint lavage (see Section 7.27, p. 257)
- valuable calves with severe joint destruction may benefit from radical surgery via arthroscopy or arthrotomy with aim of joint ankylosis

Prognosis guarded or poor unless intensive nursing is undertaken.

Discussion
Meningitis occurs in a minority of neonatal calves, usually in the first week, and is rapidly fatal. In slightly older calves septic physitis (e.g. of distal radius or distal tibia) may complicate the initial signs, and radiography then valuable. 'Joint ill' is an emergency requiring rapid control and good nursing, as well as prompt review of the possible predisposing factors.

7.18 Contracted flexor tendons

Introduction
Most frequently observed congenital anomaly in dairy breeds, and rarely acquired, congenital flexed tendons (CFT) are usually primarily in the forelegs and generally bilateral.

Signs
Mild cases have slight carpal flexion and intermittent knuckling of the fore fetlocks, then bearing weight on the dorsum of the fetlock.

More severe cases can bear weight only on the flexed fetlocks. Advanced cases, with severe contracture, are often recumbent and, when encouraged to stand, tend to fall down immediately. Such calves are usually colostrum deficient, dehydrated and very weak, having failed to suck since birth.

Palpation reveals excessive tension and tautness in both the superficial (SFT) and/or deep flexor tendons (DFT), when attempts are made to straighten the leg. No pain is evident on extension, and joint swelling is absent (compare 'joint ill' see Section 7.17, p. 238).

Treatment
- in mild congenital cases check immune status and general condition (give colostrum in first 12 hours postpartum) if doubt exists as to whether calf has taken maternal milk
- keep with dam for first 24 hours observation in well-bedded loose box or at pasture, as exercise encourages progressive correction of the milder cases of flexion of carpus and fetlock joint
- in mild case consider elongation of claw toes with piece of wood glued to sole
- in more severe case initially correct any systemic problem and consider applying splint on palmar aspect of limb: from pastern to midmetacarpus (fetlock flexion) or up to proximal radius (in carpal flexion)

- select lightweight splint material e.g. split PVC piping. Pad limb (bandage) meticulously before fitting splint. Lift calf if unable to stand up initially
- alternatively consider casting limb over padding (e.g. Lightcast), ensuring its easy removal for examination of flexion status after one to two weeks

Surgery

In severe cases of fetlock and carpal flexion (CFT) surgical correction may be attempted (see Figure 7.12).

- perform surgery in sedated calf (xylazine 0.2 mg/kg i.m.) restrained in lateral recumbency, and either IVRA or local infiltration of 2% lignocaine
- routine skin preparation along entire length of metacarpus
- make 10 cm longitudinal incision laterally over SFT and DFT in mid-metacarpal region
- carefully dissect through fascia, identifying and avoiding damage to lateral palmar digital nerve and adjacent vessels lying plantar to metacarpus both medially and laterally
- elevate SDF by inserting slightly curved Mayo scissors (see Figure 1.1, p. 3) transversely between SDF and DFT and transect SDF
- check degree of fetlock flexion again and if inadequate elevate DFT and section similarly
- finally, if necessary, section the suspensory ligament (interosseus muscle) in the proximal third of metacarpus
- close peritendinous fascia in continuous pattern with non-absorbable material, and skin with interrupted sutures
- apply light bandage and use splint if flexion still inadequately corrected by surgery and additional extension is needed, also in event of iatrogenic secondary over-extension of fetlock
- in congenital carpal flexion section of the *ulnaris lateralis* and *flexor carpi ulnaris* tendons is performed through a 7–8 cm incision, the distal commissure of which lies over the accessory carpal bone
- lightly bandage limb
- prophylactic antibiotics are not needed, but analgesics are advisable for several days (e.g. NSAID such as flunixin meglumine)
- remove splint and/or cast after 7–10 days to assess improvement

Discussion

The prognosis for CFT is good in calves with a mild deformity, i.e. sporadic knuckling of fetlocks. Severe fetlock and carpal deformaties often fail to be corrected despite the tenotomy procedures described above, flexion persists and locomotion is impossible.

Scrupulous management of splints in neonatal calves ensures avoidance of skin necrosis at potential pressure sores (see Figure 7.16).

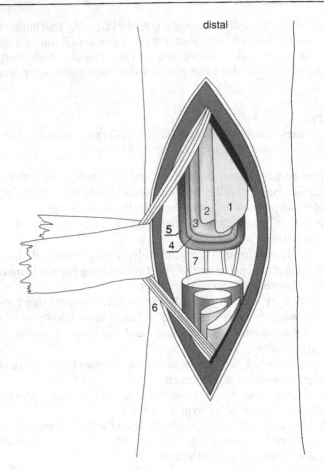

distal

Figure 7.12 Tenotomy of superficial and deep flexor tendons and suspensory ligament over left metacarpus (palmar view).
1. superficial part of superficial flexor; 2. deep part of superficial flexor; 3. deep flexor; 4. superficial part of suspensory ligament (interosseus muscle); 5. deep part of suspensory ligament; 6. medial vein, artery and nerve; 7. palmar metacarpal veins. (From Dirksen, Gründer & Stöber, 2002.)

7.19 Tarsal and carpal hygroma

Introduction
Synonyms: tarsal cellulitis, carpal/tarsal 'bursitis'.

Definition: firm or fluctuating swelling involving pre-carpal bursa and acquired subcutaneous bursa over lateral aspect of hock.

Incidence and aetiology: high in housed cattle on hard floors with little bedding.

Signs
- usually no lameness, no pain, and presents purely as cosmetic blemish
- sometimes skin contusion, break in integument, with seropurulent discharge and invasion by *Arcanobacterium pyogenes*
- distension of joint capsule, heat, pain and lameness indicate further localised spread.

Differential diagnosis: precarpal abscessation, septic carpitis, septic tarsitis.

Treatment and prophylaxis
- transfer to soft bedding or turn outside
- broad spectrum antibiotics in cases involving lameness and systemic signs
- do not open cavity or inject local corticosteroids (risk of gross contamination)
- check stall dimensions relative to breed, and any behavioural abnormalities which can be corrected
- surgical excision of a large non-infected carpal bursa with primary wound closure and pressure bandage is a possible and surgically hazardous procedure in clinic (not on-farm) situation, as wound breakdown commonly occurs despite good aftercare

7.20 Patellar luxation

Three forms exist:
- dorsal patellar luxation or fixation in adults; sporadic incidence
- lateral patellar luxation; congenital, uncommon
- medial patellar luxation; congenital, rare

Dorsal patellar luxation or fixation

Introduction
Temporary or permanent fixation of patella on upper part of medial femoral trochlear ridge.

Signs
- stiffness, later jerky action with leg extended caudally for longer than normal, followed by forward jerk (temporary fixation)
- action sometimes intermittent and limb may become fixed in rigid extension, dragging claws (permanent fixation)
- position evident on patellar palpation, and manual reposition possible.

Differential diagnosis: displacement of biceps femoris muscle, spastic paresis, acute gonitis.

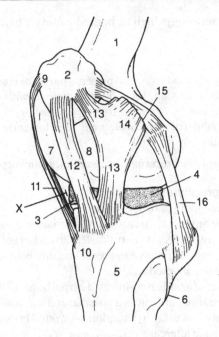

Figure 7.13 Lateral view of left stifle joint of cow.
1. femur; 2. patella; 3. and 4. medial and lateral menisci; 5. tibia; 6. fibula; 7. and
8. medial and lateral trochlear ridge; 9. patellar fibrocartilage; 10. tibial tuberosity;
11. medial straight patellar ligament (sectioned distally in patellar desmotomy);
12. and 13. middle and lateral straight patellar ligaments; 14. tendon of biceps
femoris muscle; 15. lateral femoropatellar ligament; 16. lateral collateral ligament.
X indicates site for femorotibial arthrocentesis.

Treatment

Spontaneous recovery occurs in some individuals, especially cattle at grass.
Complete recovery follows medial patellar desmotomy:

- sedate subject and produce local analgesia over lowest palpable point of
  medial straight patellar ligament (see Figure 7.13[11]), just proximal to
  insertion into tibial tuberosity
- clip and disinfect circular area 15 cm in diameter
- make vertical incision 3 cm just cranial to cranial edge of medial patellar
  ligament
- insert curved tenotome or bistoury (Hey-Groves pattern) through incision
  in vertical manner, into triangular space bounded by middle and medial
  ligaments and tibia

- turn tenotome through 90° and section ligament by short sawing movement and percutaneous pressure with finger
- withdraw tenotome in vertical position, after snapping and separation of ligament is appreciated
- appose skin edges with two simple sutures

Do **not** use disposable scalpel blade and handle, due to risk of accidental breakage and loss of blade, into periarticular area or joint. Check success of surgery immediately by observing gait; recurrence has not been reported. Surgery is best performed in standing position, though access to site may be more difficult in heavy lactating cow than in lateral recumbency.

Complications
- accidental entry into femoropatellar joint (rare)
- accidental section of middle straight patellar ligament (disastrous)
- gross iatrogenic infection of site
- severe haemorrhage

Lateral patellar luxation

Introduction
Complete or incomplete lateral displacement of patella. Femoral paralysis caused by dystocia (oversized fetus in anterior presentation, possibly 'hip-lock') may be involved in some cases, therefore check skin sensation over lateral thigh. Hypoplastic lateral trochlear ridge has been postulated but remains unproven.

Signs
- gross uni- or bilateral flexion of stifles and hocks
- limb collapses when weight is taken
- patella forms obvious bulge on lateral aspect of joint, and lateral femoral trochlear ridge is clearly palpable
- manipulative replacement sometimes possible

Differential diagnosis:

- femoral paralysis, in which a secondarily induced lateral patellar luxation may occur, but in which a discrete loss of skin sensation and quadriceps atrophy is evident (neonatal, following dystocia)
- quadriceps femoris muscle rupture, which is rare and accompanied by swelling
- gonitis, with evidence of increased synovial fluid and other joint signs
- distal femoral epiphyseal (supracondylar) separation with limb malalignment and crepitus

Treatment
- joint overlap operation: joint capsule incised medial to patella and closed by vertical mattress sutures in overlap procedure
- if patella fails to remain in trochlear groove, split fascia of thigh dorsally from patella
- create new medial patellar ligament by suturing patellar cartilage and femoral periosteum and fascia, followed by imbrication of joint capsule medially by simple interrupted absorbable sutures

Medial patellar luxation

Introduction and signs
- rare congenital condition
- complete or incomplete, permanent or intermittent
- limb flexed with patella freely moveable
- manual reposition sometimes possible

Treatment
Lateral capsular overlap procedure (see above). Prognosis is poor.

7.21 Spastic paresis

Introduction
Definition: progressive condition characterised by contraction of gastrocnemius and related calcanean tendons and muscle bellies, leading to severe over-extension of hock.

Predisposition: upright stance; certain breeds (e.g. Friesian, Aberdeen Angus) have hereditary predisposition.

Aetiology: an over-active stretch reflex is present in the gastrocnemius, with over-stimulation or lack of inhibition of motor neurons. Electromyogram (EMG) studies indicate increased electrical activity in the gastrocnemius muscle, and to a lesser extent in other muscles. CSF studies have suggested an extra-pyramidal dopaminergic central disorder.

Signs
- first seen typically at two to nine months old, rarely congenital or older animals
- initially unilateral, later often bilateral hindlimb stiffness and increasing rigidity with heel bulbs raised off ground
- intermittent backward jerking of limb, later over-extension of hock
- raised tail head with occasional upward movement
- leg is readily and painlessly flexed manually, but immediately resumes over-extended position

- weight increasingly transferred to forequarters, and progressive atrophy of hindquarters
- radiographic tarsal joint changes after several months are characteristic of chronic over-extension

Differential diagnosis: dorsal luxation of patella, septic or aseptic gonitis or tarsitis, fracture dislocation of calcaneus, joint-ill, luxation of biceps femoris muscle.

Treatment

Tenotomy of gastrocnemius tendon or tibial neurectomy. Tenotomy often only temporarily successful in young calves (< 9 months).

Tenotomy (see Figure 7.14)
- operate on standing calf under local analgesia
- shave and disinfect area over calcanean tendon 10 cm proximal to point of hock
- incise skin 6 cm long vertically over caudal aspect of tendon
- identify gastrocnemius tendon and either section transversely, or remove 2 cm portion

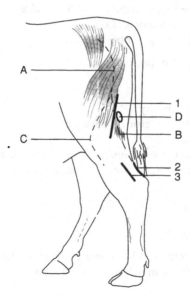

Figure 7.14 Neurectomy and tenotomy sites for alleviation of spastic paresis.
1. incision site for tibial neurectomy; 2. incision for caudal approach for gastrocnemius tenectomy; 3. incision for lateral approach for gastrocnemius tenectomy; A. sciatic nerve; B. tibial nerve; C. peroneal nerve; D. popliteal lymph node.

- section through half of transverse diameter of adjacent superficial digital flexor tendon
- suture skin

The effect is a marked dropping of hock on weight-bearing. Some operated calves develop fibrous union in operated area, leading to recurrence 1.5–3 months later. Guarded prognosis.

Neurectomy of tibial nerve (see Figure 7.14)
Tibial nerve supplies gastrocnemius muscle.

- identify and mark on skin the groove between two heads of biceps femoris in standing calf
- operate in lateral recumbency under epidural or GA
- make aseptic surgical approach between two heads of biceps femoris muscle; popliteal lymph node is useful landmark adjacent to both tibial and peroneal nerves
- insert wound retractor
- identify the two nerves by electrical nerve stimulator (e.g. cattle goad); tibial nerve causes digital flexion and hock extension, while peroneal causes digital extension and hock flexion
- remove 2 cm length of main trunk of tibial nerve, as precise identification of gastrocnemius branches is difficult or impossible
- suture subcutaneous tissues and skin
- encourage limited exercise for two weeks

Good prognosis follows this neurectomy.

Complications
- continuing muscle atrophy
- temporary or persistent peroneal paralysis
- wound breakdown
- gastrocnemius rupture in heavy cattle one to five days after neurectomy, possibly due to overstretching of denervated muscle

7.22 Hip luxation

Introduction
Relatively common condition in younger cows (two to five years), femoral head usually moving in cranial and dorsal direction.

Signs
- standing animal is obviously lame
- limb appears shortened (in dorsal dislocation)
- characteristic asymmetry of greater femoral trochanters

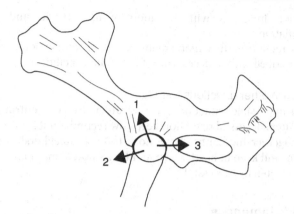

Figure 7.15 Lateral view of left half of bony pelvis showing directions of hip (femoral head) dislocation or luxation:
1. craniodorsal (frequent); 2. cranioventral; 3. caudoventral into obturator foramen (palpable).

- possible rotation of femoral shaft appreciable
- crepitus on femoral abduction and rotation
- rectal examination may reveal femoral head in obturator formen (caudal ventral dislocation) or cranial to pubic brim (cranial and ventral) (see Figure 7.15).

Aetiology: severe trauma (e.g. fall, knock, slipping), secondary to obturator paralysis postpartum, or to hypocalcaemia.

Differential diagnosis: obturator paralysis, pelvic fracture, fracture of femoral neck, fracture of femoral greater trochanter.

Treatment
Manipulative or surgical reduction within 24 hours has a good prognosis. The method varies with the direction of dislocation.

Craniodorsal dislocation
Attempt reduction under deep sedation and muscle relaxation (guaifenesin 5%)

- cast with dislocated limb uppermost
- fix cow to immoveable object (e.g. stanchion, tree trunk)
- place heavy block between ground and medial femoral region to act as fulcrum
- simultaneously exert force in three directions: longitudinally by rope on digit of affected limb, medially by pressure on lateral aspect of stifle, and caudally on greater trochanter by operator's hands

- relaxation improves with duration of anaesthesia and prolonged manipulation
- open reduction with reinforcement of the acetabular joint capsule has been described with a success rate of 75% (clinic facilities).

Dislocation in other directions (see Figure 7.15)
Difficult or impossible reduction. Success rate of 30% for ventral luxation is claimed. After successful reduction keep cow recumbent for one to two days by tying together hindlimbs above hock to avoid likelihood of immediate recurrence, and keep in box for two months. Surgical methods of reduction and fixation often unsuccessful.

7.23 Stifle lameness

Introduction
The stifle is often the site of non-digital joint problems in adult cattle, specifically degenerative arthritis. Bilateral spontaneous osteoarthritis may sometimes be inherited in Holstein and Guernsey cattle, possibly through a single autosomal recessive gene. Patellar abnormalities are discussed elsewhere (see Section 7.20, p. 243).

Injuries may primarily affect:

- cranial, and rarely also the caudal cruciate ligament (rupture)
- menisci, usually medial (tear)
- articular cartilage of femoral condyle, especially medial (erosion)

The intimate relationship of these structures in a major weight-bearing joint explains the speed of secondary changes.

Signs and gross pathology of traumatic gonitis
- sudden onset of relatively severe lameness
- increased synovial fluid (joint capsule easily appreciated) and periarticular swelling
- pain and crepitus in stifle on manual flexion, extension, rotation, abduction, and adduction
- instability possibly evident in stifle on medial to lateral movement of os calcis with limb elevated
- synovial fluid (sterile puncture between medial and middle straight patellar ligaments) blood-tinged, some debris, no evidence of sepsis (see Table 7.1)
- rapid development of secondary damage following primary injury: severe erosion of cartilage, eburnation of bone, meniscal cartilaginous erosion, tearing and displacement, extensive periarticular fibrosis, secondary cruciate rupture

Treatment

Cull cases with cranial cruciate rupture except for purebred or valuable cattle where surgery may be attempted in a surgical clinic. In other conditions ensure absolute rest and systemic anti-inflammatory drugs for seven to ten days. Prognosis is poor.

7.24 Nerve paralysis of limbs

Five different nerves may occasionally be paralysed. The aetiology, signs, diagnosis, treatment and prognosis of obturator, peroneal, femoral, sciatic and radial paralysis are summarised in Table 7.7 page 252.

7.25 Limb fractures

Introduction

Fractures can affect many bones in cattle including:

- ribs – commonest bovine fracture
- tail – likewise common, and insignificant
- vertebrae – potentially fatal
- pelvis – dystocia, involving separation of pubic symphysis in heifers; trauma (e.g. during oestrus or passing through narrow gateway) resulting in fracture of *tuber coxae*

Limb fractures involving the appendicular skeleton, including epiphyseal separation in growing stock, are relatively common.
Specific features in cattle include:

- economic considerations: in many cattle salvage may be preferable to prolonged recovery period
- humane handling and recovery facilities: often sparse compared to those for other species, and may affect proposed treatment

Long bone fractures

Common sites in descending order of incidence: metatarsus, metacarpus, tibia, femur, radius/ulna, humerus.

Treatment

- external fixation: plaster of Paris (Gypsona®, Cellona®), polyurethane resin on polyester-cotton fabric (Baycast®, Cuttercast®) or fibreglass (Deltalite®, Scotchcast®), fibreglass on cotton base (Crystona®) or polyester polymer on cotton base (Hexcelite®), hanging splint with per-cutaneous fixation (Thomas splint or walking cast), see Figure 7.16

Table 7.7 Common paralyses of cattle.

	Obturator	Peroneal	Femoral	Sciatic	Radial
Aetiology	Dystocia	Falls, postpartum recumbency	Large neonatal calves unique stretch injury (dystocia)	Pelvic fractures	Prolonged lateral recumbency in GA; some humeral fractures
Signs	Often bilateral Hindlimbs abducted	Knuckling of fetlock	Partial weightbearing possible lateral patellar luxation, discrete quadriceps atrophy in one week	Non-weightbearing	Dropped elbow, knuckled fetlock, inability to advance limb
Diagnosis	Confirmatory signs of pelvic injury	Loss of skin sensation dorsally	Specific neurogenic atrophy, possibly limited skin analgesia	Loss of all distal skin sensation	Signs and some sensory loss over elbow laterally
Differential	Adductor rupture, separated pubic symphysis	Dorsal patellar luxation	Femoral, pelvic fractures hip dislocation (dystocia) muscle tendon rupture	Femoral fracture	Humeral fracture, elbow infection
Treatment	In all five forms of paralysis only supportive treatment can be given: soft bedding, non-slip surfaces, analgesics, and vitamin B complex injection				
Prognosis	Good, but risk of a secondary hip dislocation in struggling (keep hocks together in 'figure of 8' rope until able to stand)	Good	Guarded	Guarded	Good if not sectioned (humeral fracture ends)

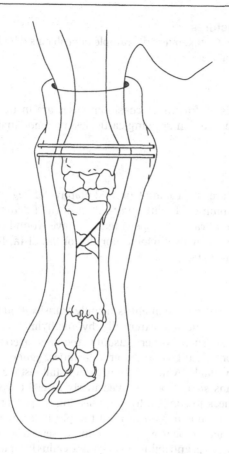

Figure 7.16 Walking cast for stabilisation of a comminuted metacarpal (MCIII/IV) fracture with two pins inserted into distal radius.

- internal fixation: steel or titanium plates and screws, Kirschner-Ehmer device, transfixation pins with overlaid resin bridge holding pins (see Figure 7.16), Kuntscher nail, Steinmann nail (and possibly multiple parallel nails or 'stack pinning').

Common problems of bovine long bone fractures:

- high incidence of comminuted fractures, often grossly displaced
- frequently compound with gross contamination
- often severe muscular contraction, increasing difficulty in manipulative reduction

For methods of internal and percutaneous fixation, reader should refer to standard textbooks (see Further reading, pp. 259–260).

Tibial shaft fractures

This fracture type is taken as an example of problems which are liable to be met in attempts at treatment.

Incidence

Common long bone fracture, occasional cases are in neonates, traumatised by dam, others are in growing cattle, less common in mature cows and bulls.

Signs

Most fractures are in proximal or mid-diaphyseal region of tibial shaft, oblique and comminuted, with over-riding of the fracture ends. Most are closed. Compound fractures (open) tend to have wound on medial aspect. Lameness is severe, with obvious mobility of the distal limb and marked crepitus at fracture site.

Treatment

While the preferred management is usually transfixation pinning (3 proximal, 3 distal), connected externally by methylmethacrylate side bars or fibreglass cast, such surgery usually requires referral to a specialist clinic where controlled traction, sterile facilities, general anaesthesia and radiology are available. Animals should have stall rest for some weeks. The transfixation pins should be removed in six to eight weeks, ideally after radiographic check to confirm fracture healing is appropriate. Minor complications include suppuration around the pin holes. Major problems are continuing inability to bear weight, leading to severe lateral bowing of the contralateral hind leg, and failure of adequate callus formation.

Thomas splint cast management is not easy. The device must be 'made to measure' and well-padded over the major pressure points in the inguinum. Some cattle find it difficult to stand up initially with such a splint.

The use of a resin or fibreglass cast alone in an attempt to immobilise a mid- or proximal diaphyseal tibial fracture is doomed to failure as it is impossible to immobilise the stifle joint. This does not apply to fractures of lower limb bones (e.g. metatarsus/metacarpus), where external immobilisation with a cast is usually the treatment of choice.

Immediate immobilisation on-farm for transport to clinic

It is imperative to minimise movement at the fracture site during transport, as a simple fracture can so easily be converted into a compound disaster. A Robert Jones bandage, with lateral support proximally to the level of the *tuber coxae* in tibial fractures, is a good insurance policy against further iatrogenic injury.

Physeal separation (Salter-Harris fracture)

Introduction

Since affected tissue is the cartilage of the growth plate, separation is a more accurate term than fracture. Majority occur at 0–12 months old. Common sites include proximal and distal femur, proximal tibia, and distal metatarsus and metacarpus. The last two forms have recently increased in incidence as a result of forced traction in beef breed heifers with dystocia caused by absolute fetal oversize. The latter has a poor prognosis due to severe bruising and failure of blood to reach the separated epiphysis, which has no nutrient artery. Osteomyelitis is common sequel.

Signs and treatment

- slight or no displacement causes mild lameness, slight crepitus, swelling, and little or no abnormal mobility
- marked displacement causes considerable movement and crepitus at fracture site, and little weight-bearing, though pain may not be marked
- prognosis is good following reduction and immobilisation of fracture under sedation or anaesthesia of lower limb
- poor prognosis for external coaptation in proximal tibial and any femoral epiphyseal separation with marked displacement, due to the difficulty of adequate immobilisation
- if external immobilisation is impossible, the choice is referral to specialist clinic or immediate slaughter

7.26 Use of acrylics and resins in orthopaedic problems

Introduction

These products are useful in several ways:

- external fixation of long bone fractures
- to fill in cracks in hoof wall, giving support to potentially weak area
- to bind toes together (as alternative to wire) to reduce post-operative trauma to interdigital space following resection of hyperplastic tissue, and secondly to prevent dorsiflexion of digit in which deep flexor tendon action has been lost by rupture or surgical resection of tendon
- in digital prosthetic blocks

Application to long bone fractures

Comparable strength of product is important in selection: (least → greatest) plaster of Paris (Johnson & Johnson), resin plaster, thermoplastic polymers (Hexcelite®), resin-bonded fibreglass (Deltalite®, Johnson, Scotchcast®, 3M). Weight of cast is important in considering desirability of limited mobility for patient. Strength:weight ratio is more favourable for resin and fibreglass products than plaster. Products may also be used in layers, e.g. plaster of Paris overlaid with thin layer of fibreglass, which is also water-resistant.

Padding (Soffban®, bandages) should be covered with brightly-coloured flexible bandage (Vetrap®) before being overlaid with fibreglass resin casting material (Dynacast Pro®). The bright colour ensures that when it is time to remove the cast, the correct depth of cut can be seen when using the electrical cast saw.

Padding (muslin bandage 3 mm thick) should be applied in growing animals. External supports should immobilise joints immediately proximal and distal to fractured long bone, e.g. midshaft fracture of metacarpus should have the cast from the proximal radius to the hoof.

Cases of recent compound fractures of metacarpus/metatarsus in small calves should be cleansed very thoroughly, and treated by external coaption with a cast or external fixator with sidebar for treatment by irrigation of the infected focus. Cows with compound fractures of > 6 hours duration should be managed with an external fixator, or be culled, depending on value of animal. Drains should *never* be left in place in such areas due to danger of ascending infection. Compound fractures carry a poor prognosis.

Application to digit

Surfaces should be prepared before application of resin

- clean off all loose foreign material
- trim any excessive horn from toe, bearing surface, and wall
- apply fat solvent with swabs
- groove bearing surface to increase contact area of resin (grinder very useful and efficient)
- dry hoof with electric hair drier in damp weather
- carefully observe manufacturer's instructions regarding mixing of product (hoof compound, Technovit [Heraeus-Kulzer]).

Other wooden blocks are produced by Demotec (Nidderau, Germany), plastic block (e.g. Podobloc®) by Agrochemica, Bremen.

Note that nowadays a wood shoe is usually put on to resin surface (which acts as glue), elevating digit further and saving much resin material, (e.g. Technovit). In using resin to elevate digit, material should be applied as an enveloping moccasin slipper to include part of abaxial and axial wall and toe. In one type of shoe (Cowslip®, Giltspur) which functions as a slipper – two lengths, 110 mm and 130 mm are available – the liquid resin is placed within the shoe before its application.

In cold weather place container of hardener in warm water before use. Also use hair drier (or even electric paint-stripper on 'low' setting) to cure resin.

Other uses of resin include the maintenance of toes in close apposition, and for protection of a vertical fissure or sandcrack. A specific indication is treatment of fracture of the distal phalanx (see Section 7.10f, pp. 217–219). The resin material is extremely hard-wearing but can shatter on sudden impact with stone or brick. After four to six weeks it can be removed by hammer blows, or with electric grinder.

Metal and rubber shoes are also available to be nailed onto claw.

7.27 Antibiotherapy of bone and joint infections

Management
Treatment of osteomyelitis, bone abscess and septic arthritis with systemic antibiotics presents major problems due to difficulties of penetration, especially of discrete foci of purulent infection walled off from vascularised tissues. Appropriate choice (see also Table 1.12 p. 46), based on first examination, is as follows:

- streptococci: penicillin G, ceftiofur
- salmonellae: oxacillin ampicillin
- penicillinase-producing staphylococci: cephalosporin and trimethoprim and sulpha, ceftiofur
- gram negative organisms: aminoglycosides (streptomycin, kanamycin, neomycin, gentamicin)
- *Arcanobacterium*: amoxycillin

Treatment of acute osteomyelitis should be continued for two to three weeks after signs of lameness have disappeared. In chronic conditions of bones and joints specific indications for surgery include abscessation with a fistulous track into bone marrow, or subperiosteal sequestrum formation.

Surgery
Joint drainage procedures for cattle include:

- needle aspiration (usually inadequate)
- joint lavage through separate entry and exit portals (14 gauge needles)
- distension irrigation
- arthrotomy with and without synovectomy.
- arthroscopy

Surgery has been more effective than medical treatment for septic arthritis in cattle.

Delay in treatment reduces the prognosis by allowing further periarticular fibrosis and articular damage. Systemic and intra-articular administration of antimicrobial agents is indicated. If given intra-articularly, the dose rate should not exceed the once daily systemic dose rate. Treatment should start before sensitivity results are available. Ceftiofur Na is often the selected drug and should be given for two weeks after the joint has returned to normal function. In cases where the primary source of infection is the umbilicus, surgical resection is indicated (see Section 3.13, p. 127).

If antibiotics and synovial aspiration do not bring improvement within 36 hours, joint lavage is indicated:

- insert two or more 14 gauge needles aseptically into different joint pouches with animal under deep sedation or light anaesthesia (e.g. ketamine) before intra-articular fibrin has developed (very acute cases)
- infuse lavage solution (polyionic) under pressure to distend joint synovial membrane and break down adhesions
- periodically block outflow needle to promote distension
- one to four litres usually used in septic joint
- arthroscopy permits large ingress and egress portal, larger volumes of solution (eight to twelve litres per session), removal of fibrin and visual inspection of the articular cartilage
- when inflammatory process becomes chronic, remove fibrin clots and abnormal synovial membrane by arthroscopy
- alternatively perform arthrotomy, and protect open joint from environmental contamination by a sterile bandage until the incision heals by secondary intention

Appendices

1 Further Reading

Anderson, D.E. ed., (March 2001) 'Lameness', *Veterinary Clinics of North America: Food Animal Practice*, 17, 1, 1–223 (multiple topics)

Andrews, A.H. ed., (2000) *The Health of Dairy Cattle*: Chapter 10 'Internal cattle building design and cow tracks' (J. Hughes); Chapter 11 'Dairy farming systems: husbandry, economics and recording' (D. Esslemont & M.A. Kossaibati), Oxford: Blackwell Scientific

Blowey, R.W., & Weaver A.D., (2003) *Color Atlas of Diseases and Disorders of Cattle*, 2nd edn. London: Mosby

Brumbaugh, G.W., (ed.) (November 2003) 'Clinical Pharmacology update' in *Veterinary Clinics of North America: Food Animal Practice*, 19, 3, 55–726 (multiple topics)

Cox. J.E., (1987) *Surgery of the Reproductive Tract in Large Animals*, 3rd edn. University of Liverpool Veterinary Field Station, Neston, Wirral (clinical notes, detailed surgical anatomy, line drawings)

Dirksen, G., Gründer H.D., & Stöber, M., (2002) *Innere Medizin und Chirurgie des Rindes*, 4th edn. Berlin: Blackwell (German 'bible', formerly Rosenberger)

Dyce, K.M., & Wensing, C.J., (1971) *Essentials of Bovine Anatomy*, Philadelphia: Lea & Febiger

Dyce, K.M., Sack, W.O., & Wensing, C.J., (1987) *Textbook of Veterinary Anatomy*, Philadelphia: W.B. Saunders

Espinasse, J., Savey, M., Thorley, C.M., *et al.*, (1984) *Colour Atlas on Disorders of Cattle and Sheep Digits: International Terminology*, Paris: Point Vétérinaire

Fubini, S.L., & Ducharme, N.G., eds, (2004) *Farm Animal Surgery*, Philadelphia: W.B. Saunders

Greenough, P.R., & Weaver, A.D., (1997) *Lameness in Cattle*, 3rd edn., Philadelphia: W.B. Saunders

Hall, L.W., & Clarke, K.W., (1991) *Veterinary Anaesthesia*, 9th edn. London: Baillière Tindall

Hickman, J., Houlton, J., & Edwards, G.B., (1997) *Atlas of Veterinary Surgery*, 3rd edn. Oxford: Blackwell

Kersjes, A.W., Nemeth, F., & Rutgers, L.J.E., (1985) *Atlas of Large Animal Surgery*, Baltimore: Williams & Wilkins (excellent colour photographs)

Leipold, H.W., Huston, K., & Dennis, S.M., (1983) Bovine congenital defects, *Adv. Vet. Sci. & Comp. Med.*, 27, 197–271

McDaniel, B.T., & Wilk, J.C., (1990) 'Lameness in dairy cattle' in *Proceedings of British Cattle Veterinary Association 1990–1991* (from VI Symposium on disorders of the ruminant digit, Liverpool, July 1990) 66–80. (Inheritance of conformation of bovine digit and related longevity of dairy cows).

National Office of Animal Health Ltd. (NOAH), Compendium of Data Sheets for Animal Medicines 2005 (UK)

Noakes, D.E., (1997) *Fertility & Obstetrics in Cattle*, 2nd edn. Oxford: Blackwell Science

Noakes, D.E., Parkinson, T.S., & England, G.C.W., (2001) *Arthur's Veterinary Reproduction and Obstetrics*, 8th edn. London & Philadelphia: W.B. Saunders

Pavaux, C., (1983) *A Colour Atlas of Bovine Visceral Anatomy*, London: Wolfe

St. Jean, G., (ed.), 'Advances in Ruminant Orthopedics' in Veterinary Clinics of North America: Food Animal Practice, 12, 1–298 (March 1996) (multiple topics)

Toussaint Raven, E., (1985) *Cattle Foot Care and Claw Trimming*, Ipswich, UK. Farming Press (Dutch method of trimming)

Tyagi, R.P.S., & Singh, J., (1993) *Ruminant Surgery*, Delhi: CBS Publishers and Distributors (p. 484, paperback, includes camel and buffalo)

Veterinary Pharmaceuticals and Biologicals (VPB), 2001–2002 12th ed., Veterinary Healthcare Communications, 8033 Flint St., Lexena, KS 66214 (index of drugs and US manufacturers and suppliers)

Westhues, M., & Fritsch, R., (1964) *Animal Anaesthesia*, Vol. 1 *Local Anaesthesia*, Bristol: Wright (details of nerve blocks e.g. retrobulbar p. 83 pudic pp. 174–179)

Whitlock, R.H., *et al.*, (1976) *Proceedings of the International Conference of Production Diseases of Farm Animals*, 3rd edn. Wageningen, The Netherlands

Wolfe, D.F., & Moll, H.D., (1999) *Large Animal Urogenital Surgery*, 2nd edn. Baltimore & London: Williams & Wilkins (penile surgery, ovariectomy)

Youngquist, R.S., ed., (1997) *Current therapy in large animal theriogenology*, Philadelphia: W.B. Saunders (pp. 429–430 ovariectomy techniques)

2 Abbreviations

ABPI	Association of British Pharmaceutical Industry
AI	artificial insemination
ALT/SGPT	alanine aminotransferase/serum glutamin-pyruvic transaminase
AST/SGOT	aspartate aminotransferase/serum glutamic-oxaloacetic transaminase
b.i.d.	*bis in die* (2 times/day)

BP	British Pharmacopoeia
BVD/MD	bovine viral diarrhoea/mucosal disease
BWG	British wire gauge
CCF	congestive cardiac failure
CCP	corpus cavernosum penis
CNS	central nervous system
Co	coccygeal
CSF	cerebrospinal fluid
ECF	extracellular fluid
ECV	extracellular volume
EDTA	ethylene diamine-tetra-acetic acid
EMG	electromyogram
FARAD	Federal Animal Residue Avoidance Databank
FG	French gauge
GA	general anaesthesia
HS	hypertonic saline
i.m.	intramuscular
i.v.	intravenous
L	lumbar
LDA	left displaced abomasum
mEq	milliequivalent
MRL	Maximum Residue Limit
NOAH	National Office of Animal Health
NSAID	non steroidal anti-inflammatory drug
PCV	packed cell volume
PDS	(monofilament) dioxanone
PGA	polyglycolic acid
PM	postmortem
PVC	polyvinylchloride
RDA	right displaced abomasum
RTA	right torsion of abomasum
S	sacral
SARA	sub-acute ruminal acidosis
s.c.	subcutaneously
SCC	squamous cell carcinoma
SGOT	see AST
SGPT	see ALT
T	thoracic
TA	tunica albuginea
t.i.d.	*ter in die* (3 times/day)
TMR	total mixed rations
USDA	United States Department of Agriculture
USP	United States Pharmacopeia
vCJD	new variant Creutzfeldt-Jakob disease

3 Useful addresses

This short reference list is divided into:

- instrument makers and suppliers
- manufacturers and suppliers of suture materials, needles, dressing, etc.
- legal and professional bodies, press, and farming and breed societies

Drug houses are omitted since the list would be unwieldy, and their addresses are more readily available elsewhere.

Each list is subdivided geographically into the UK, North America, and others.

Instrument makers and suppliers

UK

Alfred Cox (Surgical) Ltd., Edward Rd, Coulsden, Surrey (01668 2131)

Arnolds Veterinary Products, Ltd., Cartmel Drive, Harlescott, Shrewsbury, SY13 SJ (01743 44 1632, fax 01743 462 111)

Becton Dickinson Vacutainer Systems, 21 Between Towns Road, Cowley, Oxford (01865 748 844)

Brookwick Ward & Co. Ltd., 8 Shepherds Bush Road, London W6 7PQ (0870 1118610, fax 0870 1118609), www.brookwick.com

Centaur Services, Centaur House, Torbay Road, Castle Cary, Somerset BA7 7EU (01963 350005) www.centaurservices.co.uk (Trucutliver biopsy)

Genusexpress (formerly Veterinary Drug Co.) (veterinary wholesalers) Common Road, Donnington, York, YO19 (01904 487 487, fax 01904 487 611)

Holborn Surgical Instrument Co., Dolphin Works, Margate Rd, Broadstairs, Kent CT10 2QQ (0843 61418)

Medichem International, P.O. Box 237, Sevenoaks, Kent, TN15 OZJ (01732 763 555, fax 01732 763 530), email: info@medichem.co.uk

Surgical Systems Ltd., 5 Lower Queens Road, Clevedon, North Somerset, BS21 6LX, email: david@surgicalsystems.freeserve.co.uk www. surgical.systemsltd.co.uk

North America

American Medical Instrument Corp., 133–14 39th Ave, Flushing, NY 11354 (212 359 3220)

Baxter Healthcare Corp., Pharmaceutical Divn., Valencia, CA (cat. no 9135S Tru-cut biopsy needle)

Becton Dickinson, Sandy, Utah, UT 84070 (catheters)

Dandy Products, 3314 Route 131, Goshen OH 45122

Ethicon Inc., Route 22, Somerville, NJ 08876

Haver-Lockhart Laboratories, P.O. Box 390, Shawnee Mission, KS 66201

Ideal Instruments, 401 North Western Ave, Chicago, IL 60612

I-STAT Corporation, East Windsor, New Jersey 08520

Jorgensen Laboratories, 1450 Van Buren Ave, Loveland, CO 80538 (800 525 5614), www.jorvet.com, email: info@jorvet.com

Lane Manufacturing Co., Denver, CO (K-R spey instrumentation)

Linde (Cryosurgery), 270 Park Ave, New York, NY 10017

V. Mueller, Division of American Hospital Supply Co., 6600 W. Touhy Ave, Chicago, IL 60648

NASCO Farm & Ranch, 901 Janesville Ave., Fort Atkinson, WI 53538-0901

Parks Medical Electric Inc., 19460 SW Shaw, Aloha, OR 97007

Pitman Moore Surgical Instruments Division, P.O. Box 344, Washington Crossing, NJ 08560

Shamrock Scientific Speciality Systems, Inc., 34 Davis Drive, P.O. Box 143, Bellwood IL 60104

Storz Instrument Co., 3365 Tree Court Industrial Boulevard, St Louis, MO 63122

United States Surgical Corporation, Norwalk, CT 06850 (Autosuture TA-90, stapling instrumentation)

US Surgical, Tyco Health Care, Norwalk, CT 06850

University of Saskatchewan, Engineering Dept., Sasakatoon, Canada S7N 5B4 (liver biopsy trocar)

Vet. Surgical Resources, Darling, MD 21034

Willis Veterinary Supply, Chamberlain, SD 57325 (Willis ovariectomy instrument)

Other

Aesculap Werke AG, 7200 Tüttlingen, West Germany (specialist veterinary instruments)

AMICO GmbH, D7200 Tüttlingen, P.O. Box 65, Trossinger Str. 7, West Germany (subsidiary of American Medical Instrument Corp.)

Barbot-Génia, 5 rue des Clouzeaux, Parc de la Vertone 44120 (0240302417, fax 0240031471) www.genia.fr email: sjournal@genia.fr

Concept Pharmaceuticals Pvt. Ltd., 159 C.S.T. Road, Santacruz (East), Bombay 400-098, India (veterinary instruments)

Coveto, Avenue Louis Pasteur 85607 Montaigu Cedex, France (02 51 48 80 88) www.coveto.fr

Crepin Sarl, 29 avenue de Saint-Germain des Noyers, Z1 BP 77402, Saint-Thibaud des Vignes, France (01 64 30 01 33, fax 01 64 30 40 73) www.crepin.fr

Equipement Vétérinaire: (anesthesie) Zone Industrielle Rue de I'Aube, 51310 Esteray, France (03 26 42 50 15, fax 03 26 42 50 16) email: minerve.equipvet @online.fr

General Surgical Co., 1541 Bhagivath Palace, P.O. Box 1745, Chaudni Chowk, Delhi 110006, India (veterinary instruments)

H. Hauptner, Kuller Str. 38-44, Postfach 220134, 5660 Solingen, West Germany (02122 50075) (specialist veterinary instrument maker and retailer)

S. Jagdish & C., 12/21 West Patel Nagar, New Delhi 110008, India (instruments)

Jorgen Kruuse Denmark, DK-5290, Marslev, Denmark (459 951511)

Medvet, Ludwig Bertram GmbH, Postfach 644, Spielhagenstr. 20, 3000 Hanover 1, Germany (0511 812081) (specialist bovine instruments, protective clothing)

Manufacturers and suppliers of suture materials, needles, dressings, etc.

UK

Arnolds Veterinary Products, Ltd., Cartmel Drive, Harlescott, Shrewsbury, SY13 TB (01743 441 632 fax 01743 462 111)

Becton Dickinson Vacutainer Systems, 21 Between Towns Road, Cowley, Oxford (01865-748 844)

Berk Pharmaceuticals Ltd, St Leonards House, Eastbourne, East Sussex BN21 3YG (01323 641144)

Brookwick Ward & Co. Ltd., 8 Shepherds Bush Road, London W6 7PQ (0870 1118610, fax 0870 1118609), www.brockwick.com

Centaur Services, Centaur House, Torbay Road, Castle Cary, Somerset BA7 7EU (01963 350005), www.centaurservices.co.uk

Cryoproducts, Wass Lane, Sotby, Market Rasen, Lincs, LN8 5LR (01507 343091, fax 01507 343092)

Davis & Geck, Cyanamid of GB Ltd, Fareham Rd, Gosport, Hampshire PO13 0AS (01329 236131)

Davol International Ltd, Clacton-on-Sea, Essex

Duncan Flockhart & Co. Ltd. 700 Oldfield Lane North, Greenford, MX UB6 0HD (01 422 2331)

eBiox Ltd, Enterprise House, 17 Chesford Grange, Woolston, Warrington, WA14SY (0800 612 0431), email: sales@ebioxvet.co.uk, www.ebioxvet.co.uk

Ethicon Ltd., 14–18 Bankhead Av., Sighthill, Edinburgh (0131 453 5555, fax 0131 453 6011) (suture manufacturers)

Genusexpress (formerly Veterinary Drug Co.) (veterinary wholesalers), Common Road, Donnington, York, YO19 5RU (01904 487 487, fax 01904 487 611)

Holborn Surgical Instrument Co., Dolphin Works, Margate Rd, Broadstairs, Kent CT10 2QQ (01843 61418)

Johnson & Johnson Ltd, Brunel Way, Slough, Berks SL1 1XR (01753 31234)

Kruuse UK Ltd, 14a Moor Lane Industrial Estate, Sherburn-in-Elmet, N. Yorks LS25 6ES (01977 681523, fax 01977 683537), email: kruuse.uk@kruuse.com, www.kruuse.com

Medichem International, P.O. Box 237, Sevenoaks, Kent, TN15 0ZJ (01732 763 530), email: info@medichem.co.uk

Pal Wear Ltd, P.O. Box 144, Protection Works, Oadby, Leics LE2 5LW (disposable gloves, overshoes, oversleeves, trousers, coveralls, etc.)

Portek Ltd., Bleaze Farm, Old Hutton, Cumbria LA8 0LU (01539 722628, fax 01539 741282) email: info@portek.co.uk (cow blocks and glue)

Reckitt & Coleman, Pharmaceutical Division, Dansom Lane, Hull HU8 7DS (01482 26151)

Smith & Nephew Healthcare, Healthcare House, Goulton Street, Hull HU3 4DJ (01482 222200, fax 01482 222211)

Surgical Systems Ltd., 5 Lower Queens Road, Clevedon, North Somerset, BS21 6LX email: david@surgicalsystems.freeserve.co.uk, www.surgicalsystemsltd.co.uk

Teisen Products Ltd., Bradley Green, Worcs B96 6RP (01527 821488, fax 01527 821665) (hoof tape, teat bandage, tar hoof dressing)

North America

American Giltspur Inc., P.O. Box 49433, Sarasota, FL34230 ('Cowslips', 3 sizes)

AVSC (American Veterinary Supply Company), P.O. Box 9002, Knickerbocker Ave., Bohemia, NY 11716

American Hospital Supply Co., 6600 W. Touhy Ave, Chicago, IL 60648

Baxter Healthcare Corp., Pharmaceutical Div., Valencia, CA (cat. no. 9135S Tru-cut biopsy needle)

Becton Dickinson & Co., Lincoln Park, NJ07035, also Sandy, Utah, UT84070 (catheters)

Davis & Geck, American Cyanamid Company, Pearly River, New York, NY 10965

Davol Inc. (Johnson & Johnson Company) (1 800 332 2761), www.vetsurgicalexcellence.com

Dispomed, 1325 DeLanuadiere Joliette, Quebec J6E 3N9, Canada

Ethicon Inc., Route 22, Somerville, NJ 08876

Haver Lockhart Laboratories, P.O. Box 390, Shawnee Mission, KS 66201

Johnson & Johnson, 501 George St, New Brunswick, NJ 08903

Jorgensen Laboratories, 1450 Van Buren Av., Loveland, CO 80538 (800 525 5614), www.jorvet.com, info@jorvet.com

Monoject Divison, Sherwood Medical, St Louis, MO 63103

NASCO Farm & Ranch, 901 Janesville Ave., Fort Atkinson, WI 52538 0901

Pfizer Animal Health, 812 Springdale Drive, Exton, PA 19341

Provet, P.O. Box 2286, Loves Park, IL 61131 (815 877 2323)

Purdue Frederick Co., 50 Washington St, Norwalk, CT (manufacturer of Betadine surgical scrub)

Sigma Chemical Co., P.O. Box 14508, St Louis, MO 63178

Smith & Nephew, Memphis, TN

Travenol Laboratories Inc., 1425 Lake Cook Rd, Deerfield, IL 60015

US Surgical, Tyco Health Care, Norwalk, CT 06850
3M Animal Care Products, St. Paul, MN 55108-1000 (resin-impregnated foam padding)

Other
Alcyon, 41 rue des Plantes, 75014 Paris (01 53 90 39 39, fax 01 53 90 39 38) www.alcyon.com
Barbot-Genia, 5 rue des Clouzeaux, Parc de la Vertone 44120 (02 40 03 24 17, fax 02 40 03 14 71) www.genia.fr email: sjournee@genia.fr
B. Braun, Melsungen, Germany (supplied by Arnolds)
B. Braun medical S.A.S., 204 avenue du Marechal Juin, F92107 Boulogne, France Cedex (01 41 10 53 00 fax 01 41 10 53099)
Centravet Materiel, ZA des Alleux, BP 360, 22106 Dinan, France (02 96 85 80 64, fax 02 96 85 80 65) email: materiel @centravet.fr
Coveto, Avenue Louis Pasteur, 85607 Montaigu Cedex, France (02 51 48 80 88) www.coveto.fr
Equipement Vétérinaire: (anesthesie) Zone Industrielle Rue de l'Aube, 51310 Esteray, France (03 26 42 50 15 fax 03 26 42 50 16) email: minerve.equipvet@online.fr
Demotec (Siegfried Demel) Brentostr. 21, D61130 Nidderau, Germany (49 6187 21200, fax 49 6187 21208); www.demotec.com (FuturaPad, Easy Bloc, claw-cutting discs)
Medvet, Ludwig Bertram GmbH, Lübeckerstr. 1, 30880 Laatzen, Germany (49) 5102 917 590, fax (49) 5102 917 599, email: mvinfo@medvet.de, www.medvet.de (cage magnet 'CAP-Super-11')
Sigma Chemie GmbH, Am Bahnsteig, D8028, Taufkirchen, Germany

Legal and professional bodies, press, and farming and breed societies

UK
British Cattle Veterinary Association, The Green, Frampton-on-Severn, Glos, GL2 7EP (01452 740816, fax 01452 741117) www.bcva.org.uk (journal 'Cattle Practice')
British Veterinary Association, 7 Mansfield St., London WIG 9NG (020 7636 6541, fax 020 7637 0620) www.vetrecord.co.uk
Commonwealth Agricultural Bureaux International (CABI), Nosworthy Way, Wallingford, Oxon OX10 8DE www: cabi-publishing.org
Dairy Farmer, CMP Information, Sovereign House, Tonbridge, Kent TN9 1RW (01732 377273) email: phollinshead@cmpinformation.com
European Medicines Agency (EMEA): www.emea.eu.int (for authorised products for ueterinary use)
Holstein UK, Scotsbridge House, Scots Hill, Rickmansworth, Herts WD3 3DB
HSE Books: Video: *Deal with the danger: safe cattle handling*, Health and Safety Executive, HSE Books, P.O. Box 1999, Sudbury, Suffolk CO10 2WA

(01787 881165, fax 01787 313995), www.hsebooks.co.uk (ISBN 07176 2512 5)

National Office of Animal Health (NOAH) Ltd., 3 Crossfield Chambers, Gladbeck Way, Enfield, Middlesex EN2 7HF (020 8367 3131), email: noah@noah.co.uk, www.noah.co.uk

RCVS Wellcome Library & Information Service, Belgravia House, 62–64 Horseferry Rd., London SW1P 2AF (020 7222 2021, fax 020 7222 2004, email: library@rcvs.org.uk www.rcvslibrary.org.uk

Veterinary Defence Society Ltd., 4 Haig Court, Parkgate Estate, Knutsford, Cheshire WA16 8XZ

Universities Federation for Animal Welfare (UFAW), The Old School, Brewhouse Hill, Wheathampstead, Herts, AL4 8AN, UK (01582 831818, fax 01582 831414) www.ufaw.org.uk (quarterly *Animal Welfare* journal)

North America

American Association of Bovine Practitioners (AABP), P.O. Box 1755, Rome GA 30162 1755 www.aabp.org email: aabphorg@aabp.org (706 232 2220, fax 706 232 2232)

American College of Veterinary Surgeons, 11N. Washington St., Suite 720, Rockville, MD 20850 www.acvs.org email: acvs@acvs.org (301 610 20 00, fax 301 610 0371)

American Veterinary Medical Association, 1931 N. Meacham Rd, Suite 100, Schaumburg, IL 60173 4360 www.avma.org (1 847 925 8070, fax 1 847 925 1329)

AVMA Professional Liability Trust, email: richard. Shirbroun@avmaplit.com (800-228-7848 ext. 4669) or rodney.johnson@avmaplit (ext. 4645)

Bovine Practitioner, 3404 Live Oak Lane, Stillwater OK 74075, USA

Center for Veterinary Medicine, USDHHS, 7519 Standish Place, Rockville, MD 20855-0001 (307 827 3800 or 1 888 INFO FDA)

Cornell University Online Consultant: www.vet.cornell.edu/consultant/consult.asp from College of Veterinary Medicine, Cornell University, Ithaca, NY 14853 6401 (607 253 3000, fax 607 253 3701)

FARAD enquiries: FARAD@ncsu.edu or FARAD@ucdavis.edu or www.farad.org

Food Safety & Inspection Service, USDA, Washington, DC 20250 www.fsis.usda.gov (202 720 7025, fax 202 205 0158)

FDA/CVM: drugs: 888-FDA-VETS (888 332 8387)

Food Animal Residue Avoidance Databank (FARAD): www.farad.org; (888 USFARAD (919) 829 4431 or (916) 752 7505)

Hoof Trimmers Association Inc., 4312 Wild Fox, Missoula, MT 59802-3607 (866 615 4663, fax 406 543 1823), www.hooftrimmers.org/ (quarterly newsletter)

USDA Meat & Poultry hotline: 800 535 4555

USDA National Animal Health Monitoring Systems (NAHMS), Fort Collins, CO 80523

VPB Veterinary Pharmaceuticals and Biologicals, 12th Edition 2001–2 Veterinary Healthcare Communications, 8033 Flint St., Lenexa, KS66214 (913 492 4300), www.vetmedpub.com (drugs, manufacturers etc)

Other

European College of Veterinary Surgeons (ECVS) Office, University of Zürich, Faculty of Veterinary Medicine, Equine Hospital, Winterthurerstr 260, CH8057 Zürich, Switzerland (41 1 635 8404 or 41 1 313 0383, fax 41 1 313 0384) email: ecvs@vetclinics.unizh.ch www.ecvs.org (monthly *Veterinary Surgery*)

Federal Veterinary Office, Schwarzenburgstr. 161, CH-Bern Switzerland (www.bvet.admin.ch)

Federation of Veterinarians of Europe (FVE), 1 Rue Defacqz, B-1000 Brussels, Belgium www.fve.org email: info@fve.org (32 2 533 7020; fax 32 2 537 28 28)

Société Francaise de Buiatrie, BP 11 F-31620 Castelnaud'estrefonds, France (05 62 14 04 50, fax 05 62 14 04 69) email: buiatrie@wanadoo.fr e.claire@wanadoo.fr www.e-claire.fr (rubrique SFB)

Swissmedic., Erlachstr. 8, CH-3000, Bern 9, Switzerland (equivalent to FDA) (www.swissmedic.ch)

World Association for Buiatrics Secretariat, Dr. G. Szenci, Secretary General, Szent Istvan University, Faculty of Veterinary Science, P.O. Box 2, H1400 Budapest, Hungary www.buiatrics.com email: oszenci@univet.hu

4 Conversion factors for old and SI units

		Multiplication factors		
	Old units	Old uniits to SI units	SI units to old units	SI units
RBC	millions/mm^3	10^6	10^{-6}	$\times 10^{12}$/l
PCV	%	0.01	100	1/l
Hb	g/100 ml	None	None	g/dl
WBC	thousands/mm^3	10^6	10^{-6}	$\times 10^9$/l
Total serum protein	g/100 ml	10	0.1	g/l
Albumin	g/100 ml	10	0.1	g/l
Bilirubin	mg/100 ml	17.1	0.0585	μmol/l
Calcium	mg/100 ml	0.25	4.008	mmol/l
Chloride	mEq/l	None	None	mmol/l
Creatinine	mg/100 ml	88.4	0.0113	μmol/l
Globulin	g/100 ml	10	0.1	g/l
Glucose	mg/100 ml	0.0555	18.02	mmol/l
Inorganic phosphate	mg/100 ml	0.323	3.1	mmol/l
Magnesium	mg/100 ml	0.411	2.43	mmol/l
Potassium	mEq/l	None	None	mmol/l
Sodium	mEq/l	None	None	mmol/l
Urea	mg/100 ml	0.166	6.01	mmol/l

Index